SERIES I

PHLEBOTOMY
TECHNICIAN
TEXTBOOK

THEORY AND PRACTICAL FUNDAMENTALS

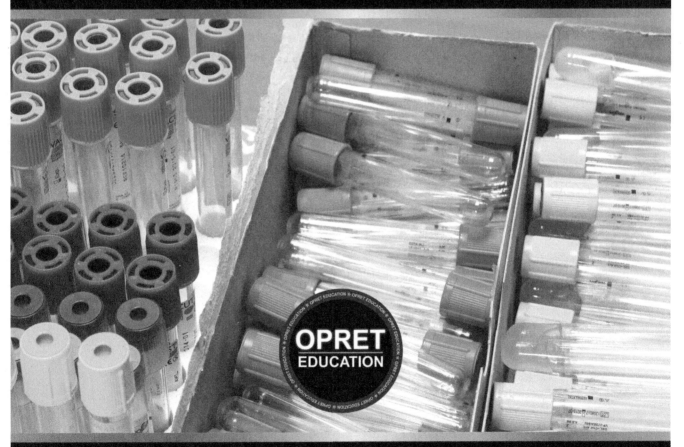

OPRET EDUCATION

PHLEBOTOMY TECHNICIAN TEXTBOOK
THEORY & PRACTICAL FUNDAMENTALS
(Series I)
ISBN: 978-1-944471-99-6
COPYRIGHT © OPRET Education

OPRET Education
Our Publications & Resources for Educational Training

www.OPRETEducation.com

Chapter 3: Medical Terminology

Chapter 4: Phlebotomy Equipment & Supplies

Chapter 5: Phlebotomy Clinical Skills

Chapter 6: Phlebotomy Fundamental Essentials

APPENDIX

CHAPTER 1: SECTION 1

INTRODUCTION TO PHLEBOTOMY & INFECTION CONTROL

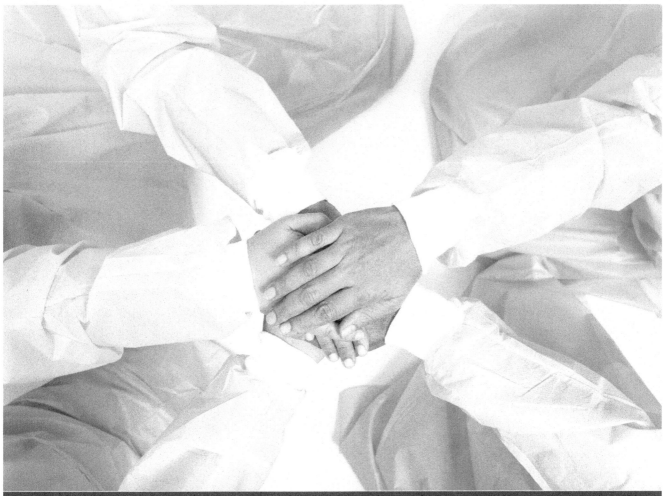

LEARNING OBJECTIVES

At the end of this chapter the student will be able to describe:

- Occupational Safety and Health Administration (OSHA)
- What type of hazards do healthcare workers face?
- Healthcare safety hazards
- Latex allergy and prevention
- Chain of infection
- Mode of transmission
- Identifying infectious patients
- Breaking the chain of infection
- Hand hygiene
- Personal protective equipment
- Standard precautions
- What are blood borne pathogens?

INTRODUCTION

Phlebotomy is a procedure of drawing blood by cutting into the vein, the first part of the word phlebotomy "Phleb" means vein, the second part of the word "tomy" means cut. A phlebotomist is a professional performing the procedure of drawing blood through different methods. The main role of the phlebotomist is to safely perform the procedure and collect the specimen (whole blood, serum or plasma) by techniques like venipuncture or dermal puncture. Additional roles may include; testing, appropriate packaging, and transporting samples collected. The sample drawn by the phlebotomist are submitted for medical screening, blood donation, research purposes, etc.

There are two main methods by which the blood sample are drawn:

1. Venipuncture: by means of cutting through a vein by a needle
2. Dermal Puncture: by means of cutting the skin layer by a lancet

Duties of a Phlebotomist may include:

- Drawing blood from patients.
- Talking to the patients and donors to decrease the level of anxiety and nervousness before having their blood drawn.
- Performing proper patient identification for appropriate labeling.
- Labeling the specimen for screening or processing.
- Entering the required patient information electronically or manually.
- Assembling, maintaining and keeping track of inventory for equipment and supplies required to perform the phlebotomy procedure.
- Performing procedures to obtain results as requested.
- Selecting the correct color tubes (with the correct additive) to draw blood for requested blood specimens.
- Explaining the procedure to the patient before performing it.
- Preparing the patient for the procedure.
- Following and demonstrating the standards of asepsis.
- Following and demonstrating standard and universal precautions.
- Performing venipuncture.
- Performing dermal puncture.
- Educating patients on the post-procedure wound care.
- Packaging and mailing or storing collected specimens for the laboratory.

- Maintaining phlebotomy log.

TRAINING

ROUTE 1:

Phlebotomists usually enter the phlebotomy occupation with a certificate from a phlebotomy program. Programs for phlebotomy are available from various community colleges, vocational schools, private career schools or technical schools. These programs usually take less than 1 year to complete and lead to a certificate or diploma. The program consists of classroom and laboratory components which include instructions in anatomy, physiology, phlebotomy equipment, theory and clinical skills of phlebotomy.

ROUTE 2:

Phlebotomists may enter the occupation with a high school diploma and receive on the job training to become a trained phlebotomist.

A phlebotomist must be trained to draw blood; the training can be received by either an approved training program or trained directly by a physician, nurse or other healthcare professionals responsible for performing phlebotomy.

PROFESSIONALISM

Displaying professional in this occupation is crucial. A phlebotomist is expected to have the right skill set, proper knowledge, good judgment, and polite behavior. Patients may have a different attitude towards their blood being drawn. Therefore phlebotomist must show a high level of professionalism. A phlebotomist must make sure to follow OSHA standards.

LICENSES & CERTIFICATIONS

Depending on the state, a phlebotomist can either get certified or licensed. Certified means that the phlebotomist has met certain standards to perform the skill, however, training is the most crucial aspect of a phlebotomist's career. Various employers hire phlebotomy technicians that are certified.

American Education Certification Association provides phlebotomy technician certification exam for candidates willing to become certified.

The exam consists of two sections:

Certification Exam Section 1: Theory Exam
Certification Exam Section 2: Clinical Skills Exam

What type of exam will the candidate take?

The certification exam is a 2 PART EXAM

Part 1: Clinical Skills Exam: the candidate will have to perform the clinical skills under the supervision of a qualified evaluator. The clinical skills competency sheet will be provided by AECA.

Part 2: Theory Exam: the candidate will challenge the multiple choice exam which will test the candidate's knowledge in the respective areas of phlebotomy.

AREAS OF EMPLOYMENT

Hospitals, Physician Offices, Laboratories & Blood Banks. The staff of clinical laboratories may include:

- Pathologist
- Clinical Biochemist
- Pathologist's Assistant (PA)
- Medical Laboratory Scientist (MT, MLS or CLS)
- Medical Laboratory Technician (MLT)
- Medical Laboratory Assistant (MLA)
- Phlebotomist

LABORATORY DEPARTMENTS

Laboratory medicine is generally divided into two sections and is further subdivided:

The two sections of laboratory medicine are:

1) ANATOMIC PATHOLOGY INCLUDES
   a) Histopathology,
   b) Cytopathology, and
   c) Electron Microscopy
2) CLINICAL PATHOLOGY INCLUDES
   a) Clinical Microbiology
      i) Bacteriology
      ii) Virology
      iii) Parasitology
      iv) Immunology and
      v) Mycology
   b) Clinical Chemistry
      i) Enzymology
      ii) Toxicology
      iii) Endocrinology
      iv) Immunochemistry
      v) Electrophoresis
   c) Hematology and Coagulation
   d) Cytogenetics
   e) Reproductive Biology

OCCUPATIONAL SAFETY AND HEALTH ADMINISTRATION (OSHA)

The Occupational Safety and Health Act (OSH Act) allows Occupational Safety and Health Administration (OSHA) to issue workplace health and safety regulations. These regulations include limits on chemical exposure, employee access to information, requirements for the use of personal protective equipment, and requirements for safety procedures.

OSHA's mission is to "assure safe and healthful working conditions for working men and women by setting and enforcing standards and by providing training, outreach, education, and assistance."

WHAT TYPES OF HAZARDS DO WORKERS FACE?

Healthcare workers face a number of serious safety and health hazards. This includes bloodborne pathogens, biological hazards, potential chemicals, drug exposures, waste anesthetic gas exposures, respiratory hazards, ergonomic hazards from lifting and repetitive tasks, laser hazards, workplace violence, hazards associated with laboratories, radioactive material, and x-ray hazards. Some of the potential chemical exposures include formaldehyde (used for preservation of specimens for pathology) ethylene oxide, glutaraldehyde, peracetic acid (used for sterilization) and numerous other chemicals used in healthcare laboratories.

HEALTHCARE SAFETY HAZARDS

- Biological Hazards
- Physical Hazards
- Sharps Hazard
- Chemical Hazards
- Electrical Hazards
- Fire or Explosive Hazards

PROCEDURE TO FOLLOW POST-EXPOSURE TO BLOOD

- Wash the area with water or antiseptic.
- Report to the employer.
- Document the injury.
- The employer must provide medical evaluation and follow-up.

LATEX

Latex Allergy: is a medical term used for a range of allergic reactions to the proteins present in latex. It is an allergy that may occur when coming into contact with products that contains latex.

Latex Sensitivity: Natural rubber latex can also cause irritant contact dermatitis, this is a less severe form of reaction that does not involve the immune system. Contact dermatitis may cause dry, itchy, irritated areas on the skin, most commonly on the hands. Latex-gloves induced dermatitis increases the chance of hospital-acquired infections (nosocomial infection).

Irritant Contact Dermatitis	Allergic Contact Dermatitis	Hypersensitivity
Reactions	**Reactions**	**Reactions**
Red, dry, itchy irritated areas	Itchy, red rash, small blisters	Hives, swelling, runny nose, nausea, abdominal cramps, dizziness, low blood pressure, bronchospasm, anaphylaxis (shock)

Table 1.1

WHAT IS CONTACT DERMATITIS?

Occupationally related contact dermatitis can develop from frequent and repeated use of hand hygiene products, exposure to chemicals and glove use. Contact dermatitis is classified as either irritant or allergic. Irritant contact dermatitis is common, nonallergic and develops as a dry, itchy, irritated areas on the skin around the area of contact. By comparison, allergic contact dermatitis (type IV hypersensitivity) can result from exposure to accelerators and other chemicals used in the manufacture of rubber gloves as well as from exposure to other chemicals found in a practice setting. Allergic contact dermatitis often manifests as a rash beginning hours after contact and, like irritant dermatitis is usually confined to the areas of contact.

WHAT IS LATEX ALLERGY?

Latex allergy (type I hypersensitivity to latex proteins) can be a more serious systemic allergic reaction. It usually begins within minutes of exposure but can sometimes occur hours later. It produces varied symptoms, which commonly include a runny nose, sneezing, itchy eyes, scratchy throat, hives, and itchy burning sensations. However, it can involve more severe symptoms including asthma marked by breathing difficulty, coughing spells and wheezing; cardiovascular and gastrointestinal ailments; and in rare cases, anaphylaxis and death.

RECOMMENDED POWDER-FREE GLOVES

When powdered gloves are worn, more latex protein reaches the skin. When gloves are put on or removed, particles of latex protein powder become aerosolized and can be inhaled, contacting mucous membranes. As a result, allergic health care personnel and patients can experience symptoms related to cutaneous, respiratory, and conjunctival exposure. Work areas where only powder-free, low-allergen (i.e. reduced-protein) gloves are used show low or undetectable amounts of allergies of such type.

PREVENTING LATEX REACTIONS

- Screen all patients for latex allergy.
- Be aware of some common predisposing conditions (e.g., spina bifida, urogenital anomalies or allergies to avocados, kiwis, nuts or bananas).
- Be familiar with different types of hypersensitivity (immediate and delayed) and the risks that these pose to patients and staff.
- Patients with a history of latex allergy may be at risk.
- Provide an alternative treatment area free of materials containing latex.
- Ensure a latex-safe environment or one in which no personnel use latex gloves and no patient contact occurs with other latex devices, materials, and products. Remove all latex-containing products from the patient's vicinity.
- Adequately cover/isolate any latex-containing devices that cannot be removed from the treatment environment.
- Be aware that latent allergens in the ambient air can cause respiratory and or anaphylactic symptoms in people with latex hypersensitivity.

- Frequently change ventilation filters and vacuum bags used in latex-contaminated areas.
- Be aware that allergic reaction can be provoked from indirect contact as well as direct contact. Hand hygiene, is, therefore, an essential component.
- If latex-related complications occur during or after the procedure, manage the reaction and seek emergency assistance as indicated. Follow current medical emergency response recommendations for management of anaphylaxis.

INFECTION CONTROL

- Infection control addresses factors related to the spread of infection within the health-care setting (whether patient-to-patient, from patients to staff, from staff to patients or among staff members).
- Including prevention (via hand hygiene/hand washing, cleaning/disinfection/sterilization/vaccination and surveillance).
- Monitoring/investigation of demonstrated or suspected spread of infection within a particular health-care setting (surveillance and outbreak investigation) and management (interruption of outbreaks).

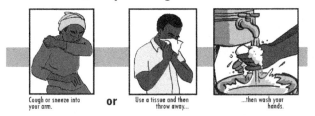

Protect Others. Protect Yourself.

Cover your cough or sneeze.

Cough or sneeze into your arm. **or** Use a tissue and then throw away... ...then wash your hands.

Stop the spread of TB, colds, and influenza.

Reference: Reference: Centers for Disease Control and Prevention

CHAIN OF INFECTION

A process that begins when an agent leaves its reservoir or host through a portal of exit, then is conveyed by some mode of transmission and enters through an appropriate portal of entry to infect a susceptible host.

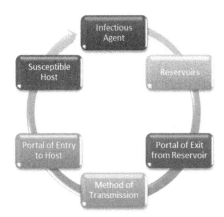

Chain of Infection Illustration 1.1

MODES OF TRANSMISSION

An infectious agent may be transmitted from its natural reservoir to a susceptible host directly or indirectly.

DIRECT

Direct contact occurs through skin-to-skin contact, kissing and sexual intercourse. Direct contact also refers to contact with soil or vegetation harboring infectious organisms. Thus, infectious mononucleosis ("kissing disease") and gonorrhea are spread from person to person by direct contact. Hookworm is spread by direct contact with contaminated soil.

Droplet spread refers to spray with relatively large, short-range aerosols produced by sneezing, coughing or even talking. Droplet spread is classified as direct because transmission is by direct spray over a few feet before the droplets fall to the ground. Pertussis and meningococcal infection are examples of diseases transmitted from an infectious patient to a susceptible host by droplet spread.

INDIRECT

Airborne transmission occurs when infectious agents are carried by dust or droplet nuclei suspended in the air. Airborne dust includes material that has settled on surfaces and become re-suspended by air currents as well as infectious particles wind-blown from the soil. Droplet nuclei are dried residue of fewer than 5 microns in size. In contrast to droplets that fall to the ground within a few feet, droplet nuclei may remain suspended in the air for long periods of time and may be blown over great distances.

Vehicles that may indirectly transmit an infectious agent include food, water, biologic products (blood) and fomites (inanimate objects such as handkerchiefs, bedding or surgical scalpels).

A vehicle may passively carry a pathogen, as food or water may carry hepatitis A virus. Alternatively, the vehicle may provide an environment in which the agent grows, multiplies or produces toxin

Vectors such as mosquitoes, flies, and ticks may carry an infectious agent through purely mechanical means or may support growth or changes in the agent. Examples of mechanical transmission are flies carrying Shigella on their appendages and flies carrying Yersinia pestis, the causative agent of plague. In contrast to biologic transmission, the causative agent of malaria or guinea worm disease undergoes maturation in an intermediate host before it can be transmitted to humans.

IDENTIFYING POTENTIALLY INFECTIOUS PATIENTS

- Facility staff shall remain alert for any patient arriving with symptoms of an active infection (e.g., diarrhea, rash, respiratory symptoms, draining wounds or skin lesions).
- If the patient calls ahead:
  - If possible have patients with symptoms of active infection come at a time when the facility is less crowded.
  - Alert registration staff ahead of time to place the patient in a private exam room upon arrival if available and follow the procedures pertinent to the route of transmission as specified by the facility.
  - If the purpose of the visit is non-urgent, patients are encouraged to reschedule the appointment until symptoms have resolved.

CONTACT PRECAUTIONS

- Applies to patients with any of the following conditions and/or diseases:
  - The presence of stool incontinence (may include patients with norovirus, rotavirus or clostridium difficile), draining wounds, uncontrolled secretions, pressure ulcers, or presence of ostomy tubes and/or bags of draining body fluids.
  - Presence of generalized rash or exanthems (rash).
- Prioritize having the patient in an exam room if they have stool incontinence, uncontrolled secretions,

draining wounds and/or skin lesions that cannot be covered.
- Perform hand hygiene prior to wearing gloves and before touching the patient.
- Personal Protective Equipment (PPE) use:
  - Wear gloves when touching the patient and the patient's immediate environment or belongings.
  - Wear a gown if substantial contact with the patient is anticipated.
- Perform hand hygiene after removal of PPE, use soap and water when hands are visibly soiled (e.g., blood, body fluids), or after caring for patients with known or suspected infectious diarrhea (e.g., Clostridium difficile, norovirus).
- Clean and disinfect the exam room accordingly.
- Instruct patients with known or suspected infectious diarrhea to use a separate bathroom, if possible clean and disinfect the bathroom before it can be used again.

DROPLET PRECAUTIONS

- Applies to patients known or suspected to be infected with a pathogen that can be transmitted by droplet route, these includes but are not limited to:
  - Respiratory viruses (influenza, parainfluenza virus, adenovirus, respiratory syncytial virus, and human metapneumovirus).
  - Bordetella pertussis.
  - For the first 24 hours of therapy (Neisseria meningitides, group A streptococcus), Place the patient in an exam room (with door closed) as soon as possible (prioritize patients who have excessive cough and sputum production); if an exam room is not available, the patient is provided a facemask and placed in a separate area as far from other patients as possible while awaiting care.
- Personal Protective Equipment (PPE) use:
  - Wear a facemask, such as a procedure or surgical mask, for close contact with the patient; the facemask should be donned upon entering the exam room.
  - If substantial spraying of respiratory fluids is anticipated: gloves, gown, and goggles (or a face shield in place of goggles) should be worn.

- Perform hand hygiene before and after touching the patient and after contact with respiratory secretions and/or contaminated objects/materials. Note: use soap and water when hands are visibly soiled (e.g. with blood and body fluids).
- Instruct patient to wear a facemask when exiting the exam room; avoid coming into close contact with other patients and practice respiratory hygiene and cough etiquette.
- Clean and disinfect the exam room accordingly.

AIRBORNE PRECAUTIONS

- Applies to patients known or suspected to be infected with a pathogen that can be transmitted by airborne route; these include, but are not limited to:
    - Tuberculosis
    - Measles
    - Chickenpox (until lesions are crusted over)
    - Localized (in immunocompromised patient) or disseminated herpes zoster (until lesions are crusted over)
- Have patient enter through a separate entrance to the facility (e.g. dedicated isolation entrance). If possible, avoid the reception and registration area.
- Place the patient immediately in an **airborne infection isolation room** (AIIR).
- If an AIIR is not available:
    - Provide a facemask (e.g. procedure or surgical mask) to the patient and place the patient immediately in an exam room with the door closed.
    - Instruct the patient to keep the facemask on while in the exam room. Change the mask if it becomes wet.
    - Initiate protocol to transfer patient to a healthcare facility that has the recommended infection-control capacity to manage the patient properly.
- PPE use:
    - Wear a fit-tested N-95 or higher-level disposable respirator. If available, don the respirator before entering the room and remove after exiting room.
    - If substantial spraying of respiratory fluids is anticipated: gloves, gown, and goggles (or a face shield in place of goggles) should be worn.

- Perform hand hygiene before and after touching the patient and after contact with respiratory secretions and/or body fluids and contaminated objects/materials. Use soap and water when hands are visibly soiled (e.g., blood, body fluids).
- Instruct patient to wear a facemask when exiting the exam room, avoid coming into close contact with other patients and practice respiratory hygiene and cough etiquette.
    - Once the patient leaves, the exam room should remain vacant for generally one hour before anyone enters. However, the adequate wait time may vary depending on the ventilation rate of the room and should be determined accordingly.
- If staff must enter the room during the wait time, they are required to use respiratory protection.

Respiratory Hygiene and Cough Etiquette

To prevent the transmission of respiratory infections in the facility, the following infection prevention measures are implemented for all potentially infected persons at the point of entry and continuing throughout the duration of the visit. This applies to any individual (e.g., patients and accompanying family members, caregivers, and visitors) with signs and symptoms of respiratory illness, including cough, congestion, rhinorrhea, or increased production of respiratory secretions.

1. Identifying Persons with Potential Respiratory Infection

- Facility staff remains alert for any persons arriving with symptoms of a respiratory infection.
- Signs are posted at the reception area instructing patients and accompanying persons to:
- Self-report symptoms of a respiratory infection during registration.
- Practice respiratory hygiene and cough etiquette (a technique described below) and wear facemask as needed.

2. Availability of Supplies:

The following supplies are provided in the reception area and other common waiting areas:

- Facemasks, tissues, and no-touch waste receptacles for disposing of used tissues.
- Dispensers of alcohol-based hand rub.

3. Respiratory Hygiene and Cough Etiquette:

All persons with signs and symptoms of a respiratory infection (including facility staff) are instructed to:

- Cover the mouth and nose with a tissue when coughing or sneezing.
- Dispose of the used tissue in the nearest waste receptacle.
- Perform hand hygiene after contact with respiratory secretions and contaminated objects/materials.

4. Masking and Separation of Persons with Respiratory Symptoms

If patient calls ahead:

- Have patients with symptoms of a respiratory infection come at a time when the facility is less crowded or through a separate entrance, if available.
- If the purpose of the visit is non-urgent, patients are encouraged to reschedule the appointment until symptoms have resolved.
- Upon entry to the facility, patients are to be instructed to don a facemask (e.g., procedure or surgical mask).
- Alert registration staff ahead of time to place the patient in an exam room with a closed door upon arrival.

If identified after arrival:

- Provide facemasks to all persons (including persons accompanying patients) who are coughing and have symptoms of a respiratory infection.
- Place the coughing patient in an exam room with a closed door as soon as possible (if suspicious for airborne transmission, refer to Airborne Precautions, if an exam room is not available, the patient should sit as far from other patients as possible in the waiting room.
- Accompanying persons who have symptoms of a respiratory infection should not enter patient-care areas and are encouraged to wait outside the facility.

5. Healthcare Personnel Responsibilities

- Healthcare personnel observe Droplet Precautions, in addition to Standard Precautions, when examining and caring for patients with signs and symptoms of a respiratory infection (if suspicious for an infectious agent spread by airborne route, refer to Airborne Precautions.
- These precautions are maintained until it is determined that the cause of the symptoms is not an infectious agent that requires Droplet or Airborne Precautions.
- All healthcare personnel are aware of facility sick leave policies, including staff who are not directly employed by the facility but provide essential daily services.
- Healthcare personnel with a respiratory infection avoid direct patient contact; if this is not possible, then a facemask should be worn while providing patient care and frequent hand hygiene should be reinforced.
- Healthcare personnel are up-to-date with all recommended vaccinations, including annual influenza vaccine.

BREAKING THE CHAIN OF INFECTION

a. Using effective hand hygiene.
b. Using personal protective equipment (PPE).
c. Isolating patients with infectious diseases.
d. Follow standard precautions.

HAND HYGIENE

- Clean hands are the single most important factor in preventing the spread of pathogens in healthcare settings.
- Hand hygiene reduces the incidence of healthcare-associated infections.
- Centers for Disease Control and Prevention (CDC) estimates that each year nearly 2 million patients in the United States get infected in hospitals, and about 90,000 of these patients die as a result of their infection.
- Widespread use of hand hygiene products that improve adherence to recommended hand hygiene practices will promote patient safety and prevent infections.
- There is substantial evidence that hand hygiene reduces the incidence of infections.
- In more recent studies healthcare-associated infection rates were lower when antiseptic hand washing was performed by personnel and went down when

13

adherence to recommended hand hygiene practices improved.

- Healthcare workers have reported several factors that may negatively impact their adherence to recommended practices including:
    a. Hand washing agents cause irritation and dryness.
    b. Inconvenient sink location.
    c. Lack of soap and paper towels.
    d. Lack of time to perform hand hygiene.
    e. Understaffing or overcrowding.

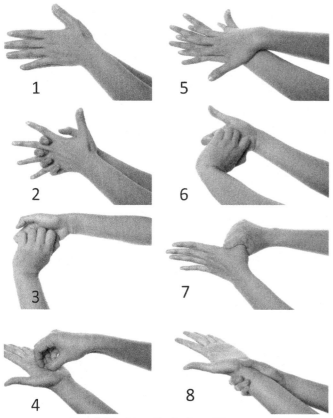

Hand Washing Technique Figure 1.1

- Lack of knowledge of guidelines/protocols, forgetfulness, and disagreement with the recommendations are also self-reported factors for poor adherence with hand hygiene.
- Hand hygiene is a general term that applies to either handwashing, antiseptic handwash, alcohol-based handrub, or surgical hand hygiene/antisepsis.
- Hand washing refers to washing hands with plain soap and water. Hand washing with soap and water remains a sensible strategy for hand hygiene in non-healthcare

settings and is recommended by CDC and other experts.

    a. Antiseptic handwash refers to washing hands with water and soap or other detergents containing an antiseptic agent.
    b. Alcohol-based handrub refers to the alcohol-containing preparation applied to the hands to reduce the number of viable microorganisms.
    c. Surgical hand hygiene/antisepsis refers to an antiseptic handwash or antiseptic handrub performed preoperatively by surgical personnel to eliminate transient and reduce resident hand flora. Antiseptic detergent preparations often have persistent antimicrobial activity.
    d. Healthcare workers should wash hands with soap and water when hands are visibly dirty, contaminated or soiled. Use an alcohol-based hand-rub when hands are not visibly soiled to reduce bacterial counts.

HAND HYGIENE: BEFORE & AFTER

- Inserting urinary catheters, peripheral vascular catheters or other invasive devices that do not require surgery.
- Before and after direct patient contact.
- After completing tasks at one patient's station before moving to another station.
- Before procedures, such as administering intravenous medications.
- Before and after contact with vascular access.
- Before and after dressing changes.
- After contact with items/surfaces at patient stations.
- Contact with a patient's skin.
- Contact with body fluids or excretions, non-intact skin and wound dressings.
- Removing gloves.

PRODUCTS USED FOR HAND HYGIENE

- Plain soap is appropriate at reducing bacterial counts, but antimicrobial soap is better and alcohol-based handrubs are the most recommended.
- Alcohol-based handrubs are less damaging to the skin than soap and water.

- The skin's water content decreases for those that use soap and water (resulting in dryer skin) as compared with those who use an alcohol-based handrub.
- Rapid access to hand hygiene materials could help improve adherence.
- Alcohol-based handrubs may be a better option than traditional hand washing with plain soap and water or antiseptic handwash because they require less time, act faster, and irritate hands less often.

HANDRUBS

- Apply to the palm of one hand, rub hands together covering all surfaces until dry.
- Application volume: based on instructions provided by the manufacturer.

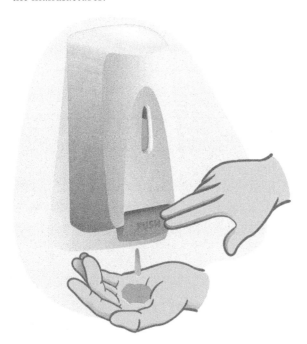

HANDWASHING

- Wet hands with water, apply soap, rub hands together for at least 15 seconds.
- Rinse and dry with a disposable towel.
- Use a towel to turn off the faucet.
- When an antimicrobial soap is used, the hands and forearms should be scrubbed for the length of time recommended by the product's manufacturer, usually 2-6 minutes. Longer scrub times (e.g. 10 minutes) are usually not necessary.
- When an alcohol-based handrub with persistent activity is used, follow the manufacturer's instructions

on the amount of product to use. Pre-wash hands and forearms with a non-antimicrobial soap and allow them to dry completely. After application of the alcohol-based product as recommended, allow hands and forearms to dry thoroughly before donning sterile gloves.

FINGERNAILS AND ARTIFICIAL NAILS

- Natural nail tips should be kept to ¼ inch in length.
- Artificial nails should not be worn when having direct contact with high-risk patients.

PERSONAL PROTECTIVE EQUIPMENT (PPE)

- "Specialized clothing or equipment worn by an employee for protection against infectious materials" (OSHA)
- OSHA issues workplace health and safety regulations. Regarding PPE, employers must:
  - Provide appropriate PPE for employees.
  - Ensure that PPE is disposed or if reusable, that PPE is cleaned, laundered, repaired and stored after use.
- OSHA also specifies circumstances for which PPE is indicated.
- CDC recommends when, what and how to use PPE.

TYPES & FUNCTIONS OF PPE

Types	Functions
Gloves	protect hands
Gowns/Aprons	protect skin and/or clothing
Masks	protect mouth/nose
Respirators	protect respiratory tract from airborne infectious agents
Goggles	protect eyes
Face shields	protect face, mouth, nose, and eyes

Types & Functions of PPE Table 1.2

SELECTING PPE

When you are selecting PPE, consider the following:

- Type of procedure to be performed.
- Amount of exposure.
- Durability and appropriateness of the PPE for the task.
- Fit (appropriate size).

GLOVES

- Wearing gloves reduce the risk of healthcare workers acquiring infections from patients, prevents flora from being transmitted from healthcare workers to patients, and reduces contamination of the hands of healthcare workers by flora that can be transmitted from one patient to another.
- Gloves should be used when Healthcare Workers (**HCW**s) have contact with blood or other body fluids.
- Gloves should be removed after caring for a patient.
- The same pair of gloves should not be worn for the care of more than one patient.
- Gloves should not be washed or reused.
- Following application of alcohol-based handrubs, hands should be rubbed together until all the alcohol has evaporated. In other words, "**Let It Dry**".
- Alcohol-based handrubs should be stored away from high temperatures or flames in accordance with the National Fire Protection Agency recommendations.

ALCOHOL-BASED RUBS

What benefits do they provide?

a. Requires less time.
b. Is more effective than standard handwashing with soap.
c. More accessible than sinks.
d. Reduces bacterial counts on hands.
e. Improves skin condition.

INSTRUCTION ON GLOVES

Most patient care activities require the use of a single pair of nonsterile gloves made of either latex, nitrile, or vinyl. However, because of allergy concerns, some facilities have eliminated or limited latex products, including gloves, and now use gloves made of nitrile or other material. Vinyl gloves are also frequently available and work well if there is limited patient contact. However, some gloves do not provide a proper fit on the hand, especially around the wrist, and therefore should not be used if extensive contact is likely to take place during patient care.

Gloves should fit the user's hands comfortably. They should not be too loose or too tight. They should not tear or damage easily. Gloves are sometimes worn for several hours and need to stand up to the task.

Type of gloves:

✓ **Glove material**: Vinyl, latex, nitrile or others.
✓ **Sterile or nonsterile**: Sterile surgical gloves are worn by surgeons and other healthcare personnel who perform invasive patient procedures. During some surgical procedures, two pairs of gloves may be worn, whereas the nonsterile gloves are worn for patient care activities as recommended.

DO'S AND DON'TS OF GLOVE USE.

1. Work from clean to dirty. This is a basic principle of infection control. In this instance, it refers to touching clean body sites or surfaces before touching the heavily contaminated areas.
2. Limit opportunities for "touch contamination" - protect yourself, others and environmental surfaces. Avoid touching any surfaces with gloves once the gloves have been in contact with a patient as this could result in a touch contamination. Surfaces, such as light switches, door and cabinet knobs can become contaminated if touched by soiled gloves.
3. Change gloves as needed. If gloves become torn or heavily soiled and additional patient care tasks must be performed, change the gloves before starting the next task. Always change gloves after use on each patient, and discard them in the nearest appropriate waste container. Patient care gloves should never be washed and used again. Washing gloves do not necessarily make them safe for reuse. It may not be possible to eliminate all microorganisms and washing can make the gloves more prone to tearing or leaking.

GOWNS OR APRONS

3 factors influence the selection of a gown or apron as PPE.

First is the purpose of use. Isolation gowns are generally the preferred PPE for clothing, but aprons occasionally are used where limited contamination is anticipated. If contamination of the arms can be anticipated, a gown should be selected. Gowns should fully cover the torso, fit comfortably over the body, and have long sleeves that fit snugly at the wrist.

Second are the material properties of the gown. Isolation gowns are made either of cotton or a spun synthetic material that dictates whether they can be laundered and reused or disposed. If fluid penetration is likely, a fluid-resistant gown should be used.

The last factor is concerned with patient risks. Clean gowns are generally used for isolation. Sterile gowns are only necessary for performing invasive procedures, such as inserting a central line. In this case, a sterile gown would serve purposes of patient and healthcare worker protection.

PPE FOR FACE

1. **Masks – protect nose and mouth**
   Masks should fully cover the nose and mouth and prevent fluid penetration. Masks should fit snugly over the nose and mouth. For this reason, masks that have a flexible nose piece and can be secured to the head with string ties or elastic are preferable.
2. **Goggles – protect eyes**
   Goggles provide barrier and protection for the eyes. Personal prescription lenses do not provide optimal eye protection and should not be used as a substitute for goggles.
3. **Face shield – protect face**
   Use face shield when skin protection, in addition to mouth, nose, and eye protection is needed. For example, when irrigating a wound or suctioning copious secretions, a face shield can be used as a substitute to wearing a mask or goggles. The face shield should cover the forehead, extend below the chin, and wrap around the side of the face.

PPE DONNING ORDER

1. Gown first
2. Mask or respirator
3. Goggles or face shield
4. Gloves

USING PPE:-

1. Keep gloved hands away from the face.
2. Avoid touching or adjusting other PPE.
3. Remove gloves if they become torn; perform hand hygiene before donning new gloves.
4. Limit surfaces and items touched.

REMOVING PPE

To remove PPE safely, you must first be able to identify what sites are considered "clean" and what are "contaminated." In general, the outside front and sleeves of the isolation gown and outside front of the goggles, mask, respirator, and face shield are considered "contaminated," regardless of whether there is visible soil.

Order of removing PPE:
1. Gloves
2. Face shield or goggles
3. Gown
4. Mask or respirator

Donning PPE

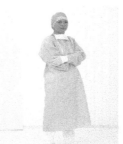

1. GOWN

2. MASK

3. GOOGLES

4. GLOVES

Removing PPE

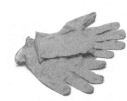

1. GLOVES

2. GOOGLES

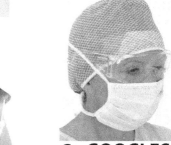

3. GOWN

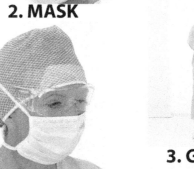

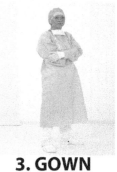

4. MASK

Order of Donning & Removing PPE Figure 1.2

Remove your PPE:

1. At the doorway, before leaving the patient room.
2. Remove respirator outside the room, after the door, has been closed.

Removing Glove Instructions:

First, using one gloved hand, grasp the outside of the opposite glove near the wrist.

Second, pull and peel the glove away from the hand. The glove should now be turned inside-out, with the contaminated side now on the inside. Hold the removed glove in the opposite gloved hand.

Third, slide one or two fingers of the ungloved hand under the wrist of the remaining glove.

Fourth, peel glove off from the inside, creating a bag for both gloves.

Finally, discard in a waste container.

Hand hygiene is the cornerstone of preventing infection transmission. You should perform hand hygiene immediately after removing PPE. If your hands become visibly contaminated during PPE removal, wash hands before continuing to remove PPE. Wash your hands thoroughly with soap and warm water or, if hands are not visibly contaminated, use an alcohol-based hand rub.

PPE DONNING & REMOVING

- Don before contact with the patient, generally before entering the room.
- Use carefully – do not spread contamination.
- Remove and discard carefully, either at the doorway or immediately outside the patient room; remove respirator outside the room.
- Immediately perform hand hygiene.

STANDARD PRECAUTIONS

Standard Precautions is an outgrowth of Universal Precautions. Universal Precautions was first recommended in 1987 to prevent the transmission of bloodborne pathogens to healthcare personnel. In 1996, the application of the concept was expanded and renamed "Standard Precautions". Standard Precautions is intended to prevent the transmission of common infectious agents to healthcare personnel, patients and visitors in any healthcare setting.

During care for patients, one should assume that an infectious agent could be present in the patient's blood or body fluids, including all secretions and excretions, except tears and sweat. Therefore, appropriate precautions, including use of PPE, must be taken. Whether PPE is needed, and if so, which type, is determined by the type of clinical interaction with the patient and the degree of blood and body fluid contact that can be reasonably anticipated and by whether the patient has been placed in isolation precautions (such as Contact or Droplet Precautions or Airborne Infection Isolation).

STANDARD PRECAUTIONS INCLUDE:

Gloves – Use when touching blood, body fluids, secretions, excretions and contaminated items; for touching mucous membranes and non-intact skin.

Gowns – Use during procedures and patient care activities. When contact of clothing/exposed skin with blood/body fluids, secretions or excretions is anticipated.

Mask and goggles or a face shield – Use during patient-care activities likely to generate splashes or sprays of blood, body fluids, secretions or excretions.

Note: For Contact Precautions – Gown and gloves are used for contact with the patient or to create an environment of care. (e.g., medical equipment, environmental surfaces)

- In some instances, these are required for entering patient's environment;
  - **For Droplet Precautions:** Use **surgical masks** within 3 feet of the patient.
  - **For Airborne Infection Isolation:** Use **particulate respirator.**

WHAT ARE BLOODBORNE PATHOGENS?

Bloodborne pathogens are infectious micro-organisms in human blood that can cause disease in humans. These pathogens include, but are not limited to, hepatitis B (HBV), hepatitis C (HCV) and human immunodeficiency virus (HIV). Needlesticks and other sharps-related injuries may expose workers to bloodborne pathogens. Workers in many occupations, including first aid team members, housekeeping personnel in some industries, nurses, and other healthcare personnel, may be at risk of exposure to bloodborne pathogens.

WHAT CAN BE DONE TO CONTROL EXPOSURE OF BLOODBORNE PATHOGENS?

In order to reduce or eliminate the hazards of occupational exposure to bloodborne pathogens, an employer must implement an exposure control plan for the worksite with details on employee protection measures. The plan must also describe how an employer will use a combination of engineering and work practice controls, ensure the use of personal protective clothing and equipment, provide training, medical surveillance, hepatitis B vaccinations, and signs and labels among other provisions. Engineering controls are the primary means of eliminating or minimizing employee exposure and include the use of safer medical devices, such as needleless devices, shielded needle devices, and plastic capillary tubes.

POST EXPOSURE TO BLOODBORNE PATHOGENS

If a healthcare worker gets stuck by a needle or other sharps or gets blood or other potentially infectious materials into their eyes, nose, mouth, or on broken skin, immediately flood the exposed area with water and clean any wound with soap and water or a skin disinfectant, if available. Report this immediately to your employer and seek immediate medical attention.

BLOODBORNE PATHOGEN STANDARDS
Requires employers to:

- **Establish an exposure control plan.** This is a written plan to eliminate or minimize occupational exposures. The employer must prepare an exposure determination that contains a list of job classifications in which workers have occupational exposure, along with a list of the tasks and procedures performed by those workers that result in their exposure.

- **Employers must update the plan annually** to reflect changes in tasks, procedures, positions that affect occupational exposure, and also technological changes that eliminate or reduce occupational exposure. In addition, employers must annually document in the plan that they have considered and begun using appropriate, commercially available, effective safer medical devices designed to eliminate or minimize occupational exposure. Employers must also document that they have solicited input from frontline workers in identifying, evaluating and selecting effective engineering and work practice controls.

- **Implement the use of universal precautions** (treating all human blood and **Other Potentially Infectious**

Materials **(OPIM)** as if known to be infectious for bloodborne pathogens).

- **Identify and use engineering controls.** These are devices that isolate or remove the bloodborne pathogens hazard from the workplace. They include sharps disposal containers, self-sheathing needles, and safer medical devices, such as sharps with engineered sharps injury protection and needleless systems.

- **Identify and ensure the use of work practice controls.** These are practices that reduce the possibility of exposure by changing the way a task is performed, such as appropriate practices for handling and disposing of contaminated sharps, handling specimens, handling laundry, and cleaning contaminated surfaces and items.

- **Provide personal protective equipment (PPE),** such as gloves, gowns, eye protection, and masks. Employers must clean, repair, and replace these equipment as required. The provision, maintenance, repair, and replacement are at no cost to the worker.

- **Make available hepatitis B vaccinations** to all workers with occupational exposure. The vaccination must be offered after the worker has received the required bloodborne pathogens training and within 10 days of initial assignment to a job with occupational exposure.

- **Maintain worker medical and training records.** The employer also must maintain a sharps injury log.

- **Make available post-exposure evaluation and follow-up** to any occupationally exposed worker who experiences an exposure incident. An exposure incident to a specific eye, mouth, other mucous membrane, non-intact skin, or parenteral contact with blood or **other potentially infectious materials (OPIM).**

- **Medical evaluation and follow-up must be at no cost** to the worker and includes:
  1. Documenting the route(s) of exposure.

2. Circumstances under which the exposure incident occurred.

3. Identifying and testing the source individual for HBV and HIV infection.

4. Collecting and testing the exposed worker's blood.

- **Use labels and signs to communicate hazards.** Warning labels must be affixed to containers of regulated waste:
  1. Containers of contaminated reusable sharps.
  2. Refrigerators and freezers containing blood or OPIM.
  3. Other containers used to store, transport, or ship blood or OPIM.
  4. Contaminated equipment that is being shipped or serviced and
  5. Bags or containers of contaminated laundry, except as provided in the standard. Facilities may use red bags or red containers instead of labels.

- **Provide information and training to workers.** Employers must ensure that their workers receive regular training that covers all elements of the standard including, but not limited to:
  1. Information on bloodborne pathogens and diseases.
  2. Methods used to control occupational exposure.
  3. Hepatitis B vaccine.
  4. Medical evaluation.
  5. Post-exposure follow-up procedures.

- **Employers must offer this training on initial assignment**, at least annually after that, and when new or modified tasks or procedures affect a worker's occupational exposure. The training must be presented at an educational level and in a language that workers understand.

Sterilization is a process that destroys or eliminates all forms of microbial life and can be carried out via physical or chemical methods. Steam under pressure, dry heat, hydrogen peroxide gas plasma, and liquid chemicals are some sterilizing agents used in healthcare facilities. When chemicals are used for destroying all forms of microbiological lives, they can be called as chemical sterilants.

METHODS OF STERILIZATION

- **Steam** is the preferred method for sterilizing critical medical and surgical instruments that are not damaged by heat, steam, pressure, or moisture.
- **Cool steam- or heat-sterilized** items before they are handled or used in the operative setting.
- Follow the sterilization times, temperatures, and other operating parameters (e.g., gas concentration, humidity) recommended by the manufacturers of the instruments, the sterilizer, and the container or wrap used, and that are consistent with guidelines published by government agencies and professional organizations.
- **Use low-temperature sterilization** technologies (e.g., EtO, hydrogen peroxide gas plasma) for reprocessing critical patient-care equipment that is heat or moisture sensitive.
- Completely aerate surgical and medical items that have been sterilized in the EtO sterilizer (e.g., polyvinylchloride tubing requires 12 hours at 50°C, 8 hours at 60°C) before using these items in patient care.
- **Sterilization using the peracetic acid immersion system** can be used to sterilize heat-sensitive immersible medical and surgical items.
- **Critical items that have been sterilized by the peracetic acid immersion** process must be used immediately (i.e., items are not completely protected from contamination, making long-term storage unacceptable).
- **Dry-heat sterilization** (e.g., 340oF for 60 minutes) can be used to sterilize items (e.g., powders, oils) that can sustain high temperatures.
- Comply with the sterilizer manufacturer's instructions regarding the sterilizer cycle parameters (e.g., time, temperature, concentration).
- Because narrow-lumen devices provide a challenge to all low-temperature sterilization technologies, and direct contact is necessary for the sterilant to be effective, ensure that the sterilant has direct contact with contaminated surfaces (e.g., scopes processed in peracetic acid must be connected to channel irrigators).

Disinfection is a process that eliminates many or all pathogenic microorganisms, except some bacterial spores. In health-care settings, most of the objects are disinfected by liquid chemicals or wet pasteurization.

Some Chemical Disinfectants are:-
- ✓ Alcohol
- ✓ Chlorine and Chlorine Compounds
- ✓ Formaldehyde
- ✓ Glutaraldehyde
- ✓ Hydrogen Peroxide
- ✓ Iodophors
- ✓ Ortho-phthalaldehyde (OPA)
- ✓ Peracetic Acid
- ✓ Peracetic Acid and Hydrogen Peroxide
- ✓ Phenolics
- ✓ Quaternary Ammonium Compounds

Factors that affect the effectiveness of both disinfection and sterilization include
1. Prior cleaning of the object
2. Type and the level of microbial contamination
3. Concentration of and exposure time to the germicide
4. Physical nature of the object
5. Presence of biofilms
6. Temperature and pH of the disinfection process
7. Relative humidity of the sterilization process.

Cleaning is the process of removing visible soil from objects and surfaces. This can be accomplished manually or mechanically using water with detergents or enzymatic products. Cleaning is an essential part of the process before high-level disinfection and sterilization are performed because soiling that remains on the surface of the instrument can interfere with the effectiveness of the processes.

DISINFECTION AND STERILIZATION GUIDELINE

Disinfection and sterilization are essential for making sure that medical instruments do not transmit infectious pathogens from patient to patient. Sterilization of all patient-care items may not be necessary. Health-care

facility policy must specifically identify, whether an item should be cleaned, disinfected, or sterilized.

TIPS TO PREVENT NEEDLESTICK INJURY

1) Use safe needle devices and needleless devices to decrease needlestick or other sharps exposure.
2) Properly handle and dispose of needles and other sharps according to OSHA's Bloodborne Pathogen Standard.
   a) Do not bend, recap, or remove contaminated needles and other sharps unless such an act is required by a specific procedure or has no feasible alternative.
   b) Do not shear or break contaminated sharps. (OSHA defines contaminated as the presence or reasonably anticipated presence of blood or other potentially infectious materials on an item or surface).
3) Have needle containers available near areas where needles may be found.
4) Discard contaminated sharps immediately or as soon as possible into appropriate containers.
   a) Sharps container should be:
      i) Closable, puncture-resistant, and leak-proof on sides and bottom
      ii) Accessible, maintained upright, and not allowed to overfill
      iii) Labeled or color-coded according to OSHA standard
      iv) Colored red or labeled with the biohazard symbol
      v) Labeled in fluorescent orange or orange-red, with lettering and symbols in a contrasting color (Red bags or containers may be substituted for labels)
5) Provide training to exposed employees atleast on an annual basis.
6) Assure that your facility meets all requirements of OSHA's Bloodborne Pathogen Standard.

TIPS TO PREVENT BACK INJURIES AND STRAINS

- Locate equipment and materials in the facility, in a manner that reduces the amount of lifting and handling as much as possible.

- Maintain clear open spaces around equipment and materials being handled. Easy access allows workers to get closer and reduces activities such as reaching, bending, and twisting.
- When lifting:
    a. Get a secure grip.
    b. Use both hands whenever possible.
    c. Avoid jerking by using smooth, even motions.
    d. Keep the load as close to the body as possible.
    e. To the extent feasible, use your legs to push up and lift the load, not your upper body or back.
    f. Do not twist your body. Step to one side to turn.
    g. Get help while moving large items, rather than lifting alone.
    h. Avoid awkward postures when carrying items.

SHARPS CONTAINER

A sharps container is a container that is filled with sharp medical instruments. Needles are dropped into the container without touching the outside of the container. Needles should never be pushed or forced into the container, as damage to the container and/or needlestick injuries may result.

WHAT IS THE NEEDLESTICK SAFETY AND PREVENTION ACT?

The Needlestick Safety and Prevention Act was signed into law on November 6, 2000. Due to continued problem of occupational exposure to bloodborne pathogens from accidental sharps injuries in healthcare and other occupational settings, Congress felt that a modification to OSHA's Bloodborne Pathogens Standard was appropriate to set forth in greater detail OSHA's requirement for employers to identify, evaluate, and implement safer medical devices. The Act also mandated additional requirements for maintaining a sharps injury log and for the involvement of non-managerial healthcare workers in evaluating and choosing devices.

HOW DOES THE "NEEDLESTICK ACT" APPLY TO OSHA'S BLOODBORNE PATHOGENS STANDARD?

The Act directed OSHA to revise its Bloodborne Pathogens Standard. OSHA published the revised standard in the Federal Register on January 18, 2001; it took effect on April 18, 2001. The agency implemented a 90-day outreach and education effort for both OSHA staff and the regulated public before beginning enforcement of the new requirements.

IMPLEMENT SAFER MEDICAL DEVICES

The 1991 standard states, "Engineering and work practice controls shall be used to eliminate or minimize employee exposure." The revision defines Engineering Controls as "controls (e.g., sharps disposal containers, self-sheathing needles, safer medical devices, such as sharps with engineered sharps injury protection and needleless systems) that isolate or remove the bloodborne pathogens hazard from the workplace."

PROCEDURE TO FOLLOW POST – EXPOSURE TO BLOOD

- Wash the area with water or antiseptic
- Report to employer
- Document the injury
- Medical evaluation and follow-up must be provided by the employer

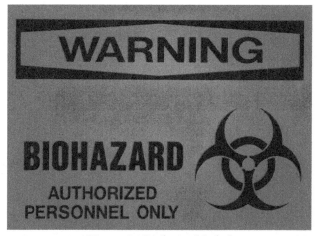

Figure 1.3 Biohazard Label

BLOODBORNE PATHOGEN SPILL GUIDELINES: PREPARING BLEACH SOLUTION
BLEACH DISINFECTING SOLUTION

1. 9 parts cool water.
2. 1 part household bleach.
3. Add the household bleach to the water.
4. Gently mix the solution.

CLEAN-UP PROCEDURE USING BLEACH SOLUTION

1. Block off the area of the spill from patrons until clean-up and disinfection is complete.

2. Put on disposable gloves to prevent contamination of hands.

3. Wipe up the spill using paper towels or absorbent material and place it in a plastic garbage bag.

4. Gently pour bleach solution onto all contaminated areas of the surface.

5. Let the bleach solution remain in the contaminated area for 20 minutes.

6. Wipe up the remaining bleach solution.

7. All non-disposable cleaning materials used such as mops, scrubs and brushes should be disinfected by saturating with a bleach solution and air dried.

8. Remove gloves and place in a plastic garbage bag with all soiled cleaning materials.

9. Double-bag and securely tie-up plastic garbage bags and discard.

10. Thoroughly wash hands with soap and water.

Reference:

1. *Centers for Disease Control and Prevention: http://www.cdc.gov/*

2. *Siegel JD, Rhinehart E, Jackson M, Chiarello L, and the Healthcare Infection Control Practices Advisory Committee, 2007 Guideline for Isolation Precautions: Preventing Transmission of Infectious Agents in Healthcare Settings http://www.cdc.gov/ncidod/dhqp/pdf/isolation2007.pdf*

3. *Occupational safety and health administration https://www.osha.gov*

4. *Allmers H, Brehler R, Chen Z, Raulf-Heimsoth M, Fels H, Baur X. Reduction of latex aeroallergens and latex-specific IgE antibodies in sensitized workers after removal of powdered natural rubber latex gloves in a hospital. J Allergy Clin Immunol 1998;102:841–846.*

5. *Leavitt JW. Typhoid Mary: captive to the public's health. Boston: Beacon Press; 1996.*

6. *Remington PL, Hall WN, Davis IH, Herald A, Gunn RA. Airborne transmission of measles in a physician's office. JAMA 1985;253:1575–7.*

7. *Guideline for Hand Hygiene in Health-care Settings. MMWR 2002; vol. 51, no. RR-16.*

8. *Guidance for the Selection and Use of Personal Protective Equipment in Healthcare Settings, Center for disease control and prevention.*

CHAPTER 1 SECTION 1
END OF CHAPTER REVIEW QUESTIONS

Question Set 1: Match the Following

Answers	Column A	Column B
	Gloves	A. may indirectly transmit an infectious agent include food, water, biologic products (blood), and fomites (inanimate objects such as handkerchiefs, bedding, or surgical scalpels).
	Sterilization	B. hives, swelling, runny nose, nausea, abdominal cramps, dizziness, low blood pressure, bronchospasm, anaphylaxis (shock).
	Gowns	C. red, dry, itchy irritated areas.
	OSHA	D. are used when touching blood, body fluids, secretions, excretions, and contaminated items; for touching mucous membranes and non-intact skin.
	Contact dermatitis	E. refers to the alcohol-containing preparation applied to the hands to reduce the number of viable microorganisms.
	Irritant Contact Dermatitis Reactions (Latex Reaction)	F. workplace health and safety regulations.
	Alcohol-based handrub	G. is a process that destroys or eliminates all forms of microbial life and can be carried out via physical or chemical methods.
	Allergic Contact Dermatitis Reactions (Latex Reaction)	H. causes dry, itchy, irritated areas on the skin, most often on the hands.
	Vehicle mode of infection transmission	I. are used during procedures and patient care activities. When the contact of clothing/exposed skin with blood/body fluids, secretions, or excretions is anticipated.
	Hypersensitivity Reactions (Latex Reaction)	J. itchy, red rash, small blisters.

Question Set 2: Essay Questions

1. What are bloodborne pathogens & what can be done to control exposure to bloodborne pathogens?
2. What is PPE? Explain types and procedure for donning and removing PPE?
3. Explain the chain of infection and various ways to break the chain of infection?
4. Explain in brief contact dermatitis?
5. Outline the cleaning up procedure for blood spills using bleach solution?
6. Explain in brief about standard precautions?
7. In brief, explain the hand hygiene procedure?
8. Explain the direct and indirect mode of transmission of infectious agents?

Question Set 3: Fill in the Blanks

1. Latex allergy generally develops after repeated exposure to products containing _____.

2. Latex allergy produces varied symptoms, which commonly include _____ nose, sneezing, _____ eyes,

   _____ throat, hives, and _____ burning sensations.

3. Chain of infection is a process that begins when an _____ leaves its _____ or host through a portal of _____,

   and is conveyed by some mode of _____, then enters through an appropriate portal of _____ to infect

   a susceptible _____.

4. Droplet spread refers to spray with relatively large, short-range _____ produced by _____,

   _____, or even _____.

5. Bloodborne pathogens are _____ microorganisms in human blood that can cause disease in humans.

Question Set 4: Multiple Choice

1. Latex allergy produces varied symptoms, which commonly include all the following except:
   ____a)   runny nose
   ____b)   sneezing
   ____c)   radiating pain
   ____d)   scratchy throat

2. Breaking the chain of infection can be done by all of the following except:
   ____a)   Using effective hand hygiene.
   ____b)   Using PPE (Personal Protective Equipment).
   ____c)   Isolating patients with infectious diseases.
   ____d)   Using HIPAA recommendations.

3. All of the followings are benefits of using alcohol-based rubs except:
   ____a)   Require less time.
   ____b)   Are less effective for standard handwashing than soap.
   ____c)   Reduce bacterial counts on hands.
   ____d)   Improve skin condition.

4. All of the following are Personal Protective Equipment except:
   ____a)   Gloves
   ____b)   Gowns
   ____c)   Sterile Pack
   ____d)   Mask

5. The correct order of donning personal protective equipment:
   ____a)   Mask or respirator, Gown first, Goggles or Face Shield, Gloves

____b)   Goggles or Face Shield, Gown first, Mask or Respirator, Gloves

____c)   Gown first, Mask or Respirator, Goggles or Face Shield, Gloves

____d)   Gloves, Gown first, Mask or Respirator, Goggles or Face Shield

6. The correct order of removing personal protective equipment:

____a)   Gloves, Face shield or goggles, Gown, Mask or respirator

____b)   Gown, Gloves, Face shield or goggles, Mask or respirator

____c)   Mask or respirator, Gloves, Face shield or goggles, Gown

____d)   Gloves, Mask or respirator, Face shield or goggles, Gown

Question Set 5: True or False (T/F)   Circle Answers

1. Infection control addresses factors related to the spread of infections within the health-care setting.

    Answer: TRUE OR FALSE

2. OSHA addresses factors related to monitoring/investigation of demonstrated or suspected spread of infection within a particular health-care setting (surveillance and outbreak investigation), and management (interruption of outbreaks).

    Answer: TRUE OR FALSE

3. Modes of transmission is a process that begins when an agent leaves its reservoir or host through a portal of exit, and is conveyed by some mode of transmission, then enters through an appropriate portal of entry to infect a susceptible host.

    Answer: TRUE OR FALSE

4. Vector transmission occurs when infectious agents are carried by dust or droplet nuclei suspended in air.

    Answer: TRUE OR FALSE

5. Droplet precautions apply to patients known or suspected to be infected with a pathogen that can be transmitted by droplet route; these include, but are not limited to respiratory viruses and bordetella pertussis.

    Answer: TRUE OR FALSE

6. Plain soap is good at reducing bacterial counts, but antimicrobial soap is better and alcohol-based handrubs are the best.

    Answer: TRUE OR FALSE

7. Artificial nails can be worn when having direct contact with high-risk patients.

    Answer: TRUE OR FALSE

8. Standard Precautions is intended to prevent the transmission of common infectious agents to healthcare personnel, patients and visitors in any healthcare setting.

    Answer: TRUE OR FALSE

9. Vectors such as mosquitoes, flies, and ticks may carry an infectious agent through purely mechanical means or may support growth or changes in the agent.

    Answer: TRUE OR FALSE

10. Infection control addresses factors related to the spread of infections within the health-care setting (whether patient-to-patient, from patients to staff, from staff to patients or among staff).

    Answer: TRUE OR FALSE

CHAPTER 1: SECTION 2
LEGAL ISSUES IN HEALTHCARE

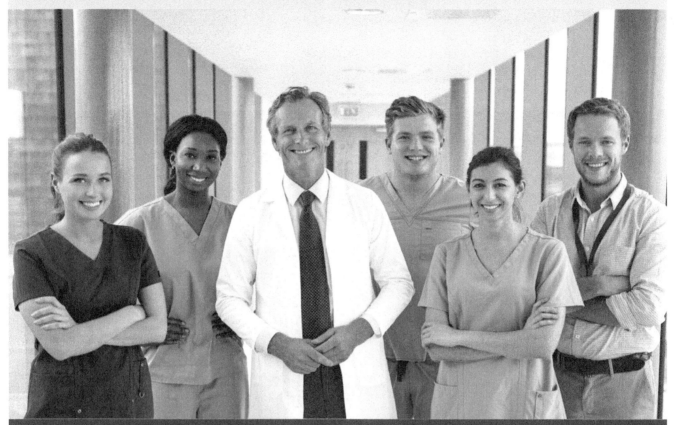

LEARNING OBJECTIVES

At the end of this chapter the student will be able to describe in brief:

Types of Laws (Civil and Criminal), with their brief descriptions, tort law

Negligence vs. malpractice

What is Standard of care?

Basic elements of negligence (duty, breach of duty, direct cause and damage)

Types of damages

      1.Special damage

      2.General damage

      3.Punitive damage

Sources of laws

Consents and its types

Patient abuse and types of abuse

Patients' rights

Patient self-determining act (PSDA)

Living will, advance directives and false imprisonment

Scope of Practice, Good Samaritan Law (GSL) and Uniform Anatomical Gift Act (UAGA)

Americans with Disabilities Act (ADA)

LEGAL ISSUES IN HEALTHCARE

Each facility has their own policies and procedures to ensure that procedures are performed as safely and correctly as possible. A standard of care should always be followed when performing a procedure. Make sure that you follow the established standard of care.

LAWS

CIVIL LAW

Deals with enforcement of all public rights (non-criminal laws). Example Tort law

TORT LAW

Torts are wrongdoings as a result of unreasonable actions of others. This may cause injury or damage to the person on whom the unreasonable action is being performed. As a result of which the injured person may take a civil action against the person or party performing the unreasonable action.

There are basically three types of torts:

1. Intentional torts
2. Negligence
3. Strict liability

Intentional Torts: action is intended to harm

- **Assault**: Threatening or causing bodily injury to another person, it may be a crime or a tort.
- **Battery**: Touching a patient without his or her consent is termed as a battery, it can either be a civil or criminal offense.
- **Defamation**: In general is a written or oral statement which causes harm to the reputation of a person or third party.
- **Slander**: A defamatory statement presented in an oral or spoken format.
- **Libel**: A defamatory statement presented in a published or written format.
- **Fraud**: Intentionally hiding the truth for unlawful gains.
- **Invasion of privacy**: Health Insurance Portability and Accountability Act of 1996 (HIPAA): Title II of HIPAA (Administrative Simplification) consists of the privacy and security rule. The main purpose of these rules is to keep a patient's health information confidential and secure.

Negligence
Unintentional Tort: actions are unintentional

Negligence: Legal cause of action resulting from a failure to exercise the care that a reasonable person would exercise in like, same or similar circumstances. Types of negligence:

- **Comparative negligence**: Both parties are involved, and the compensation depends on the contribution of the negligence, the jury decides the percentage of fault and the compensation has to be paid based on the percentage/proportion of the fault.
- **Contributory negligence**: Cases in which the plaintiffs own negligence lead to the injury.

Strict Liability:

Liability regardless of fault.

Malpractice: A substandard delivery of care by the healthcare provider causing injury to the patient.

NEGLIGENCE VS MALPRACTICE

Medical negligence occurs when a medical professional fails to do something that should have been done.

Medical malpractice means that a medical professional performed their job in a way that deviated from the accepted medical standards of care, causing injury or death. Medical malpractice is a type of negligence.

WHAT IS STANDARD OF CARE?

A standard of care can be explained as *"what would have another professional done under similar situation or circumstances."*

BASIC ELEMENTS OF NEGLIGENCE

Duty:

Is what one person owes to another. In this element, it must be proven that the defendant owed a duty to the plaintiff. A duty should first be established to prove that the defendant owed a duty to the plaintiff.

Breach of Duty:

Once established that the defendant owed a duty to the plaintiff, it must be proved that the defendant breached that duty. To prove that there was a breach of duty, the plaintiff must show that the defendant violated the standard of care or acted negligently.

Direct Cause:

The breach of duty was a direct cause of injury to the plaintiff.

Damage:

The last element in which plaintiff's injury is reviewed and compensation is sought.

TYPES OF DAMAGES

- **Special Damages** – Dollar values for damages or injury suffered by the individual (i.e. medical bills and lost wages).
- **General Damages** – No dollar value can be applied (i.e. example pain and suffering cannot be valued).
- **Punitive Damages** – Are to punish the defendant for the negligence rather than to compensate the plaintiff.

CRIMINAL LAW

The body of law that defines and governs the actions that constitute crimes.

Felony

Severe Crime, Prison for more than 1 year.

Misdemeanors

Less Severe Crime, Prison for less than 1 year.

SOURCES OF LAWS

Common Law

Law that is derived from judicial decisions instead of from statutes.

Statutory Law

Law that comes from the state and federal legislatures Statutory law consists of the laws passed by the legislature.

Administrative Law

Created by the administrative agencies for carrying out their duties and responsibilities. Administrative agencies are established to perform a specific function; they can be state or federal agencies.

CONSENT

Informed Consent

A process in which the permission is granted from the patient prior to the start of a healthcare procedure.

Expressed Consent

A type of consent in which the person expresses the permission in written or spoken words before the onset of a healthcare procedure.

Implied Consent:

A type of consent in which the permission is not expressed but rather inferred by the person's action, signs, and facts.

PATIENT ABUSE

Is any action or failure to act, which can result in physical, mental or emotional pain or injury to the patient.

- **Physical abuse**. Causes harm to a patient. Examples include pinching, punching, kicking, slapping, burning, bruising, pushing, shoving.
- **Sexual abuse**. Forcing a patient, using physical or verbal threats to indulge or participate in sexual acts.
- **Psychosocial or mental abuse**. An act of emotionally harming a patient using threats, humiliation, intimidation, isolation, insult or threatening to stop the treatment.
- **Verbal abuse**. An act of oral (yelling, calling out names, swearing, teasing) or written (insulting language) words, pictures (inappropriate pictures), or gestures that threaten, embarrasses or insults the patient.
- **Involuntary seclusion**. Involuntary isolation or separation of the patient from others.
- **Substance abuse**. Use of any drug which is illegal or lethal and can cause harm to the patient.

Abuse by others

If you find a patient being abused by anyone, report the findings to the appropriate authority. Sometimes even the patient would not know that abuse is taking place on them. **REMEMBER: IT MUST BE REPORTED.**

PATIENTS' RIGHTS

Type of Patient Right	Purpose
The right to give or withhold authorization of disclosures	The patient generally has the right to control who has access to confidential information except as otherwise provided by law. The patient needs to give specific authorization or permission to allow a third party to have access to confidential information.
The right to maintain privacy	Only those persons directly involved in the care of the patient's health problem should have access to private information. Health care workers should protect information revealed during provider health care worker encounters, including all written or electronic records of these encounters.
The right to have autonomy	Autonomy is the right of a patient to determine what will be done with his or her body, personal belongings, and personal information; this concept applies to any adult person who is mentally competent. Sometimes the right to autonomy can be overridden in the interest of protecting others who may be harmed by the patient's decisions.
The right to be given information	The patient has a right to information about his or her medical diagnosis, treatment regimen, and progress. This allows the patient to make appropriate, informed decisions about his or her health care.

Patients have the right to:
- get the best possible care
- know their rights
- refuse treatments
- refuse restraints
- review medical records
- privacy and confidentiality
- know about their health status (transfer & discharge)
- to have their visitors
- to attend support group activities

The patient-health care worker relationship is the basis for
1. Sharing information.
2. Communicating beliefs and feelings that affect care.
3. Building trust between the patient and health care worker.

Three ways to earn a patient's trust include
1. Respecting the patient's autonomy, the right of a patient to determine what will be done with his or her body, belongings, and personal information.
2. Freely providing complete and accurate information.
3. Rigorously maintaining confidentiality.

PATIENT CONFIDENTIALITY
HOW TO PROTECT
ANY SITUATION
- Confirm the patient's identity at the first encounter.
- Never discuss the patient's case with anyone without the patient's permission (including family and friends during off-duty hours).
- Never leave hard copies of forms or records where unauthorized persons may access them.
- Use only secure routes to send patient information (for example, official mail) and always mark this information confidential.
- When using an interpreter, ensure that the interpreter understands the importance of patient confidentiality.

WHEN IN AN OFFICE, CLINIC, OR INSTITUTION
- Conduct patient interviews in private rooms or areas.
- Never discuss cases or use patients' names in a public area.
- If a staff member or health care worker requests patient information, establish his or her authority to do so before disclosing anything.
- Keep records that contain patient names and other identifying information in closed, locked files.
- Restrict access to electronic databases to designated staff.

- Carefully protect computer passwords or keys; never give them to unauthorized persons.
- Carefully safeguard computer screens.
- Keep computers in a locked or restricted area; physically or electronically lock the hard drive.
- Keep printouts of electronic information in a restricted or locked area; printouts that are no longer needed should be destroyed.

WHEN IN THE FIELD

- Be discreet when making patient visits.
- Conduct patient interviews in private; never discuss the case in a public place.
- Do not leave sensitive or confidential information in messages for the patient on a door; but if a message must be left on the door, it should be left in a sealed envelope, marked confidential, and addressed to a specific person.
- Do not leave sensitive or confidential information on an answering machine that other people can access.
- Do not leave sensitive or confidential information with a neighbor or friend, and be careful not to disclose the patient's condition when gathering information on his or her whereabouts.

The Patient Self Determination Act (PSDA)

The Patient Self-Determination Act (PSDA), enacted in 1991, dictates that health care institutions must take steps to educate all adult patients on their right to accept or refuse medical care. The written information concerning advance directives must be provided to an adult individual by healthcare facilities.

The requirements of the PSDA are as follows:

- Patients are given written notice on admission. Patient rights include the rights to:
  - *Facilitate their own health care decisions.*
  - *Accept or refuse medical treatment.*
  - *Make an advance health care directive.*
- Facilities must inquire as to the whether the patient already has an advance health care directive, and make a note of this in their medical records.
- Facilities must provide education to their staff and affiliates about advance health care directives.
- Health care providers are not allowed to discriminately admit or treat patients based on whether or not they have an advance health care directive.

If an individual at the time of admission or is otherwise unable to express whether or not he/she has already executed an advance directive, information about advance directives may be given to the individual's family members.

ADVANCE DIRECTIVES: A BRIEF OVERVIEW
Living Will
A written document which includes the medical treatment the person would want and not want to receive.
Durable Power of Attorney
Gives the power (authority) to another person for making medical decisions for the patient in the event of the patient unable to take the decision himself. The name of the document used for such purpose is known as, **Protective Medical Decisions Document (PMDD)**.

Examples of what can be incorporated within the advance directive can be:

1. **Do Not Resuscitate (DNR)**
   This document indicates medical professionals not to perform CPR on the patient.
2. **Do Not Intubate (DNI)**
   This document indicates medical professionals not to perform intubation on the patient.

FALSE IMPRISONMENT
Restraint a person without proper authorization and consent. All patients have their rights and respecting their rights is crucial.

Respondeat Superior: Employers are liable for the actions of an employee within the course and scope of their employment.
Res ipsa Loquitor: Latin for "the thing speaks for itself."
Abandonment: Occurs when a healthcare personnel leaves the patient without providing the care that was needed.

Scope of Practice

Defines the procedures, actions, and processes that are permitted to perform under the licensed profession. Each state has its scope of practice for the licensed individual.

Good Samaritan Act(s)

Good Samaritan laws are laws or acts that protect those individual/s who choose to serve and tend to help others who are injured or ill. Good Samaritan laws vary from jurisdiction to jurisdiction.

Uniform Anatomical Gift Act

The Uniform Anatomical Gift Act (UAGA or the Act) was passed in the US in 1968 and has since been revised in 1987 and in 2006. "Anatomical gift" means a donation of all or part of a human body (organs, tissues, and other human body parts) to take effect after the donor's death for the purpose of transplantation, therapy, research, or education.

Americans with Disabilities Act (ADA)

The Americans with Disabilities Act of 1990 (ADA) is a federal civil rights law that prohibits discrimination against individuals with disabilities in everyday activities, including medical services. The ADA is a wide-ranging civil rights law that prohibits discrimination based on disability. It affords similar protections against discrimination to Americans with disabilities as the Civil Rights Act of 1964, which made discrimination based on race, religion, sex, national origin, and other characteristics illegal.

5 Titles of the ADA

Title I—Employment
Title II—Public entities
Title III—Public accommodations
Title IV—Telecommunications
Title V—Miscellaneous provisions

References:

a. *Washington State Legislature, Revised Code of Washington (RCW), Title 68, Chapter 68.64, Section 68.64.010*

b. *Centers for Disease Control and Prevention: http://www.cdc.gov/tb/education*

c. *Civil Rights Act of 1964 Archived 14 November 2009 at WebCite*

d. *Americans with Disabilities Act, Access To Medical Care For Individuals With Mobility Disabilities, July 2010*

e. *CFR Title 42; Chapter IV; Subchapter G; Part 483; Subpart B*

f. *The Joint Commission. The Comprehensive Accreditation Manual for Hospitals: Human Resources.*

CHAPTER 1 SECTION 2
END OF CHAPTER REVIEW QUESTIONS

Question Set 1: Essay Questions

1. Explain in brief about different types of consents?

2. Explain in brief about ADA.

3. What is the standard of care?

4. How to protect patient confidentiality?

5. What are the basic elements of negligence?

6. Explain different types of damages?

7. Summarize your findings in a case involving medical negligence.

8. Summarize your findings in a case involving medical malpractice.

9. Explain in brief Scope of Practice, Good Samaritan Act(s) and Uniform Anatomical Gift Act?

10. Explain the difference between assault and battery, give one example of each?

ANATOMY & PHYSIOLOGY

CHAPTER 2: INTRODUCTION TO HUMAN ANATOMY & PHYSIOLOGY

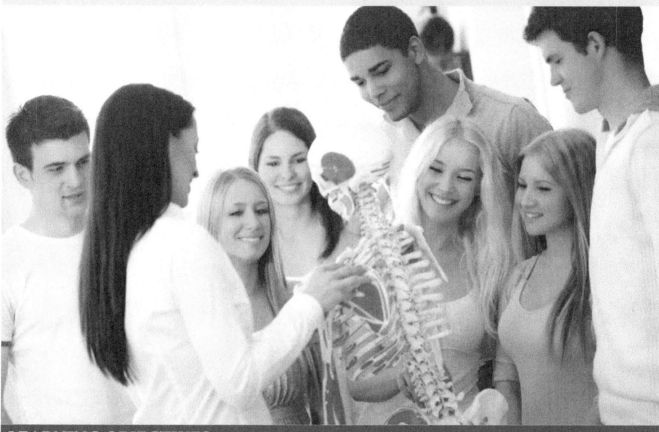

LEARNING OBJECTIVES

At the end of this chapter the student will be able to describe in brief:

Vascular system

Human Blood & Connective Tissue

Formed Elements & Proportion of Blood

Red blood cell (RBC)

White blood cells (WBC)

Platelets

Hemostasis

Blood plasma

Blood serum

Antibody and antigen

Blood transfusion and blood groups

Arterial system: Function & Structure

Venous system: Function & Structure

Capillary: Function

Veins for phlebotomy

Introduction to Integumentary system

Introduction to Heart

Introduction to Pulmonary System

Introduction to Skeleton System

Introduction to Nervous System

Introduction to Urinary System

Introduction to Digestive System

Introduction to Endocrine System

Body planes /Directional/Movement terminologies

VASCULAR SYSTEM:
HUMAN ANATOMY & PHYSIOLOGY

Anatomy, the term relates to the structure of the human body. Physiology, the term relates to the functional aspect of the human body, about how the human body functions. An example to explain the difference between anatomy and physiology would be to consider the human heart. The heart has its own parts and its components, this would be the anatomy of the heart. While how the heart functions, pumping and relaxing would be considered the physiology of the heart. Another example would be the red blood cells, also known as the RBCs. The anatomical aspect of the red blood cells would be the shape, size, components, etc. Whereas the function of the red blood cell would be the physiological aspect.

Human Blood

The human blood consists of various types of blood cells (red blood cells, white blood cells, platelets) that contains a variety of constituents. The vital function of the blood cells mainly the red blood cells is to carry oxygen and other constituents required by the tissues and on the other hand collect carbon dioxide and waste materials from the tissues and the vital function of the white blood cells is to protect the body.

The red blood cells are also known as "**Erythrocytes**", and the white blood cells are also known as "**Leukocytes**". According to the medical terminology, the terminology part "**Erythr**" means the color red, whereas the terminology part "**cytes**" means the cells. On the other hand, the terminology part "**Leuk**" means the color white, whereas the terminology part "**cytes**" means the cells. The red blood cells or the erythrocytes are abbreviated as **RBCs** and the white blood cells, or the leukocytes are abbreviated as **WBCs**. The platelets are present in fragments; their main function is to seal the injured blood vessel. They are also known as "**Thrombocytes**". The blood is mainly red in color and differs in volume due to factors such as gender, age, weight, and etc. The volume of blood is usually higher in males. The constituents of the blood also differ depending on whether the blood is in the arterial system or the venous system. If the blood is in the arterial system, it mainly consists of oxygenated blood which simply means blood that contains oxygen, while the blood in the venous system mainly consists of deoxygenated blood which simply means blood that contains carbon dioxide.

Why is blood a Connective Tissue?

The blood is a type of connective tissue. Connective tissue has the following characteristics:
1. Ground Substance
2. Fibers
3. Cells

The blood has all the above characteristics of a connective tissue.

Characteristics	Human Blood
1. GROUND SUBSTANCE	Plasma is the ground substance
2. FIBERS	Fibers
3. CELLS	Formed Elements are the cells

Table 2.1

Blood has the ground substance, plasma. It also has fibers that are proteins that assists in clotting of blood and the cells are the formed elements.

Formed Elements

There are three type's cells:

1. Erythrocytes
2. Leukocytes
3. Thrombocytes

As discussed earlier, that the red blood cells (RBCs) are also known as "**Erythrocytes**", and the White blood cells (WBCs) are also known as "**Leukocytes**" and the Platelets are also known as "**Thrombocytes**".

PROPORTION OF BLOOD

The **Plasma** in the blood is on an average about 55% of the blood, and the formed elements **form** the remaining 45% of the blood. From the 45% of the formed elements, less than 1% is the **White Blood Cells** and the **Platelets**, whereas the rest is the **Red Blood Cells.**

THE ELEMENTS OF BLOOD

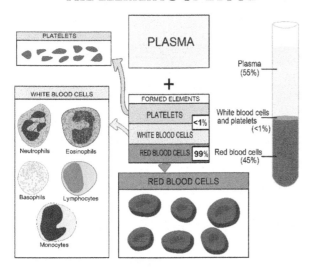

Figure 2.1

Plasma 55%	Water 90% Solutes 10%
Formed Elements 45%	Leukocytes Thrombocytes Erythrocytes

Figure 2.2

RED BLOOD CELL (RBC)

The red blood cells are the major portion of the formed elements. The shape of the red blood cell is that of a disc. It is thick at its outer end and thin towards the center. It is red in color. It consists of **hemoglobin**. Hemoglobin is the main component responsible for transporting oxygen from the lungs to the tissues and carbon dioxide from the tissues to the lungs. The hemoglobin is made up of **Heme**: iron component and the **Globin**: protein component. The heme portion of the hemoglobin can hold up to 4 oxygen molecules. There are 2 types of hemoglobin:

1. Oxyhemoglobin
2. Deoxyhemoglobin

The **oxyhemoglobin** carries oxygen molecules, whereas the **de-oxyhemoglobin** carries the carbon dioxide molecules.

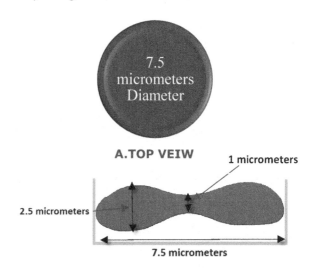

A. TOP VEIW

B. SIDE VIEW Figure 2.3

NORMAL SIZE OF RBC

Diameter: 7.5 micrometers (6.9 to 7.8 micrometers).

NORMAL RANGE OF RBC (MALE VS FEMALE)

The normal range for men is approximately **4.7 to 6.1** million cells/μl (microliter). The normal range for women is from **4.2 to 5.4** million cells/μl (microliter), according to NIH (National Institutes of Health) data.

WHITE BLOOD CELLS (WBCS)

The white blood cells are less than 1% of the 45% formed elements. They are produced in the human bone marrow. There are 5 types of white blood cells in the human blood. They are:

1. Basophils,
2. Eosinophils,
3. Neutrophils,
4. Monocytes, and
5. Lymphocytes.

Each type of the white blood cells is distinguished by the function they perform. The white blood cells number increases when required. The main function of the white blood cells is to provide immunity.

- When leukocytes **increase** in number, the condition is termed as **Leukocytosis**.
- When leukocytes **decrease** in number, the condition is termed as **Leukopenia**.

Other conditions that affect the:

1) Eosinophils are

    a) **Eosinophilia** (increase in the number of eosinophils),

    b) **Eosinopenia** (decrease in the number of eosinophils).

2) Neutrophils,

    a) **Neutrophilia** (increase in the number of neutrophils),

    b) **Neutropenia** (decrease in the number of neutrophils).

3) Basophils,

    a) **Basophilia** (increase in the number of basophils),

    b) **Basopenia** (decrease in the number of basophils).

4) Monocytes

    a) **Monocytosis** (increase in the number of monocytes),

    b) **Monocytopenia** (decrease in the number of monocytes).

5) Lymphocytes.

    a) **Lymphocytosis** (increase in the number of lymphocytes),

    b) **Lymphocytopenia** (decrease in the number of lymphocytes).

Apart from the 5 types of white blood cells, the white blood cells are also distinguished based on the presence and absence of granule.

The white blood cells that have a presence of granules are known as **granulocytes**, whereas the white blood cells that have an absence of granules are known as **agranulocytes**.

The white blood cells that are granulocytes are the:

1) Basophils
2) Eosinophils
3) Neutrophils

Remember: BEN

The white blood cells that are agranulocytes are the:

4) Monocytes
5) Lymphocytes

Conditions affecting the:

Granulocytes.

    a) **Granulocytosis** (increase in the number of granulocytes),

    b) **Granulocytopenia** (decrease in the number of granulocytes).

MORPHOLOGY OF WHITE BLOOD CELLS

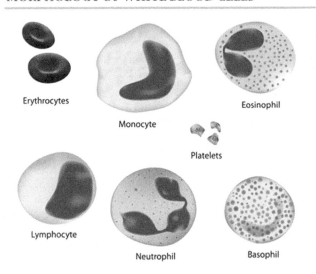

Figure 2.4

WBC TYPES	
WBC	**TYPE**
Basophils	Granulocyte
Eosinophils	Granulocyte
Neutrophils	Granulocyte
Monocytes	Agranulocyte
Lymphocytes	Agranulocyte

WBC FUNCTIONS	
WBC	**FUNCTION**
Basophils	Releases heparin and histamine. Heparin inhibits coagulation (clotting) making it possible for the other white blood cells to flow and Histamine cause vasodilation for increasing the blood flow to the area.
Eosinophils	Provide immune response against parasitic infection. They

	are also seen in response to an allergic reaction.
Neutrophils	Provides immunity by protecting the body against bacteria and fungi. They are phagocytic in nature.
Monocytes	Performs the function of phagocytes by the process of phagocytosis, however, they are less phagocytic in nature than the neutrophils. They help other white blood cells in recognizing the pathogens.
Lymphocytes	They are of 3 types: T cells, B cells, and Natural killer cells. T cells provide immunity by the release of cells such as phagocytes and proteins such as cytokines etc. B cells provide immunity by producing antibodies. Natural killer cells are activated in response to cytokines.

WBC %	
WBC	**% OF TOTAL WBC**
Basophils	0.5 -1%
Eosinophils	2 - 4%
Neutrophils	40 - 60%
Monocytes	2 - 8%
Lymphocytes	20 - 30%

Process of Phagocytosis

Phagocytosis is a process whereby an antigen is engulfed, digested and disintegrated by a phagocytic cell.

1) The process starts by the antigen coming in contact with the phagocytic cell.
2) Phagocyte-antigen adherence takes place.

3) The antigen enters the phagocytic cell, after which the antigen is engulfed forming a phagosome. The phagosome and lysosome form phagolysosome.
4) Digestion of the antigen.
5) Remains of the digestion process are expelled out of the cell in the form of debris.

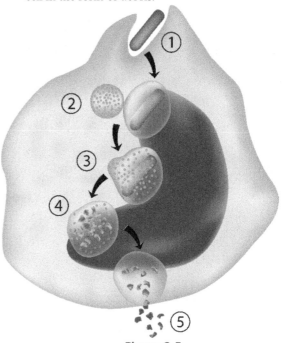

Figure 2.5

PLATELETS

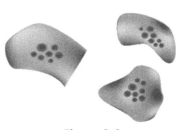

Figure 2.6

Platelets is one of the constituents of the formed elements. Their main function is to clot blood. They are colorless cells within the human blood. They are present in fragments. Platelets are also known as **thrombocytes**.

Conditions affecting the:

Thrombocytes

- **Thrombocytosis** (increase in the number of thrombocytes),
- **Thrombocytopenia** (decrease in the number of thrombocytes).

HEMOSTASIS

Hemostasis is defined as a process which causes stoppage of bleeding.

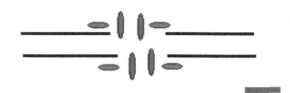

Injury of Blood Vessel

Figure 2.7B

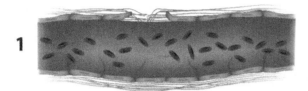

INJURED BLOOD VESSEL

1

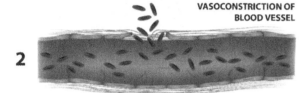

VASOCONSTRICTION OF BLOOD VESSEL

2

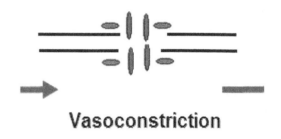

Vasoconstriction

Figure 2.7C

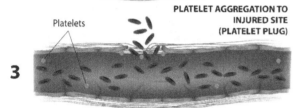

Platelets

PLATELET AGGREGATION TO INJURED SITE (PLATELET PLUG)

3

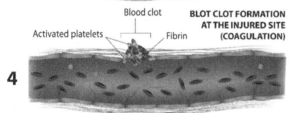

Blood clot

Activated platelets   Fibrin

BLOT CLOT FORMATION AT THE INJURED SITE (COAGULATION)

4

Figure 2.7A

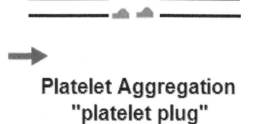

Platelet Aggregation "platelet plug"

Figure 2.7D

| blood
| subendothelial cells
| platelets

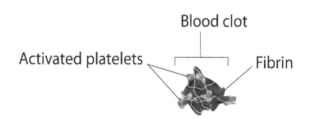

Blood clot

Activated platelets   Fibrin

Figure 2.7E Formation of a Blood Clot

STAGES OF HEMOSTASIS

1. Vasoconstriction
2. Platelet plug formation
3. Coagulation of blood

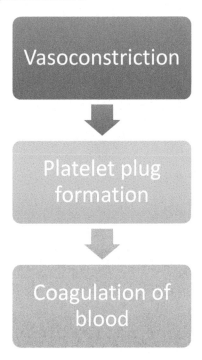

Stages of Blood Clotting

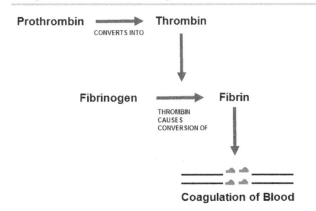

Figure 2.7F

BLOOD PLASMA

Plasma is the yellow (FLUID) portion of the blood. It is 55% of the human blood. Separating plasma from the blood can be done by obtaining blood in a blood collection tube, followed by centrifuging the tube for 15 minutes at recommended rotations per minutes in a centrifuge device. At completion, a yellow layer will be seen as a top layer in the blood collection tube. The yellow layer seen is the plasma. Using a pipette, draw the plasma and transfer it into the vial.

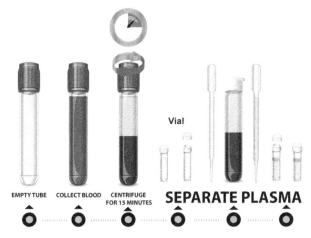

Figure 2.8 BLOOD PLASMA

BLOOD SERUM

Separating serum from the blood can be done by obtaining blood in a blood collection tube, and letting the blood to clot for 30-45 minutes, followed by centrifuging the blood collection tube for 15 minutes at recommended rotations per minutes in a centrifuge device. At completion, a yellow layer will be seen as a top layer in the blood collection tube. The yellow layer seen is the serum. Using a pipette, draw the serum and transfer it into the vial.

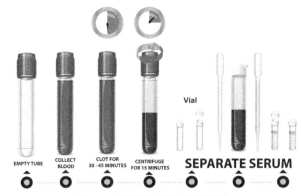

Figure 2.9 BLOOD SERUM

ANTIBODY & ANTIGEN

Antibodies are substances that are produced in the human body in response to an invading micro-organism. Another name used for antibodies is immunoglobulins. Antigens on entering the body activates the immune response which leads to the production of an antibody.

BLOOD TRANSFUSION

Blood transfusion is the procedure of transferring blood from the donor to the recipient. To transfer blood from one person to another, the compatible blood types (ABO and Rh type) needs to be transfused to avoid any complications.

Blood Groups

- ABO group
- Rhesus group

ABO BLOOD GROUPS

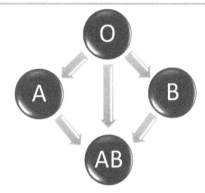

Red Blood Cell Compatibility Chart
Type O blood donors can donate blood to A, B, and AB
Types A and B blood donors can donate blood to AB
Figure 2.10

Rh

The Rh blood group is classified on the basis of whether a Rh antigen is present or absent. If the Rh antigen is present, the blood type is positive. If the Rh antigen is absent, the blood type is negative.

Blood Group A, B, AB, & O may be positive or negative depending on whether the Rh antigen is present or absent.

Blood Groups	If Rh Antigen Absent	If Rh Antigen Present
A	-A	+A
B	-B	+B
AB	-AB	+AB

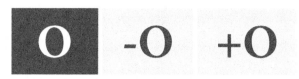

Table 2.2

If an individual has Rh antigen absent, the individual is Rh negative for that particular blood group.

If an individual has Rh antigen present, the individual is Rh positive for that particular blood group.

BLOOD TYPES (Phenotype)	'A' Group	'B' Group	'AB' Group	'O' Group
Antigens in Red Blood Cells	Antigen A	Antigen B	Antigen AB	NONE
Antibodies in Serum	antibody b	antibody a	NONE	antibody a & b
BLOOD TRANSFUSION	This blood group has Antigen A and antibody b. So a person cannot receive group B blood since the antibody b is present in this blood group. This antibody b will destroy the group B blood by considering them foreign bodies (antigens).	This blood group has Antigen B and antibody a So a person cannot receive group A blood since the antibody a is present in this blood group, This antibody a will destroy the group A blood by considering them foreign bodies (antigens).	This blood group has Antigen AB and no antibody. This group can receive blood from both group A & B since there is no antibody present.	This blood group has NO Antigen, and has antibody a & antibody B; This group cannot receive blood from both group A & B since there is antibody present against A & B. "O" also called as universal donors.

Receiver Blood Types	Donor Blood Types				
Phenotype	Antibody	A	B	AB	O
A	Anti - B	√	×	×	√
B	Anti - A	×	√	×	√
AB	NONE	√	√	√	√
O	Anti – A & Anti - B	×	×	×	√

√ : Can Receive ×: Cannot Receive

Table 2.3

HUMAN ANATOMY: INTRODUCTION TO BLOOD VESSELS (CARDIOVASCULAR)

Vessels of the circulatory system are the aorta, arteries, arterioles, capillaries, venules, veins, and vena cava.

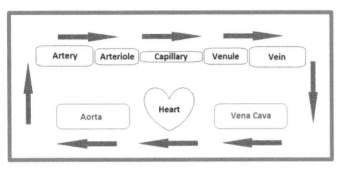

FIGURE 2.11
Direction of blood flow from the heart and back into the heart

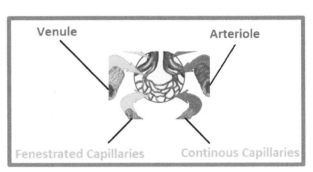

FIGURE 2.12
Venule, Capillaries, and Arteries

ARTERIAL SYSTEM

The arterial system consists of the aorta, arteries, and arterioles. Walls of the arteries are formed by three layers.

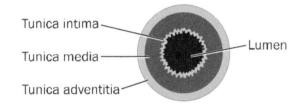

Figure: 2.13

FUNCTION:

Carries oxygenated blood (oxygen-rich blood) from the heart to the body.

STRUCTURE:

Layers of the arteries are as follows:
1. Outer tunica adventitia
2. Middle tunica media
3. Inner tunica intima

The blood flow to the organs starts by the **aorta** receiving **oxygenated blood** from the heart. Next, the aorta further narrows into an artery, the artery further narrows into an arteriole. The arteriole is the smallest vessel of the arterial system. The arteriole further continues as capillaries; capillaries function to provide oxygenated blood and nutrient to the organs and collect deoxygenated blood and waste from the organs. After this exchange has occurred at the capillary level, the capillary continues itself into a venule. The venule is the smallest vessel of the venous system. Venule further continues into a vein; the vein finally ends up into a vena cava. Vena cava is the largest veins in the human body. They are two in number namely; the **superior vena cava and the inferior vena cava**. The vena cava(s) bring **deoxygenated blood** back to the heart.

VASODILATION:

Vasodilation refers to the **increase in diameter** of the blood vessels.

VASOCONSTRICTION:

Vasoconstriction refers to the **decrease in diameter** of the blood vessels.

VENOUS SYSTEM

The venous system consists of blood vessels such as venule, vein and vena cava (superior vena cava and inferior vena cava).

FUNCTION:

Carries deoxygenated blood from the body to the heart.

STRUCTURE:

Layers of the vein are as follows:

1. Outer tunica adventitia
2. Middle tunica media
3. Inner tunica intima

CAPILLARY TYPES:

- **Continuous Capillaries**
- **Fenestrated Capillaries**

FUNCTION:

The main function of the capillaries is to give oxygen and nutrient to the tissues and collect carbon dioxide and waste from the tissues.

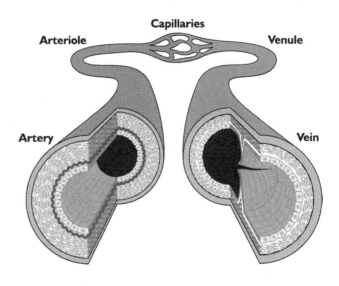

Figure 2.14

	Artery	Vein	Capillaries
Function	Carry Oxygenated Blood	Carry Deoxygenated Blood	Gives Oxygenated Blood & Collects Deoxygenated Blood

Table 2.4 DIFFERENCE BETWEEN ARTERY, VEIN, AND CAPILLARIES

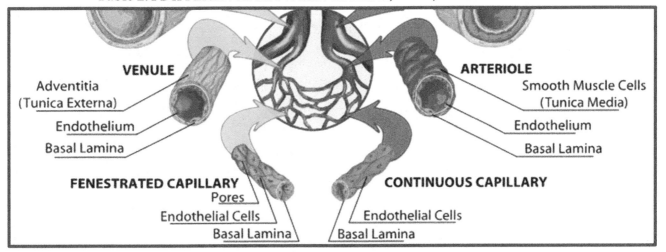

FIGURE 2.15 CONTINUOUS & FENESTRATED CAPILLARIES

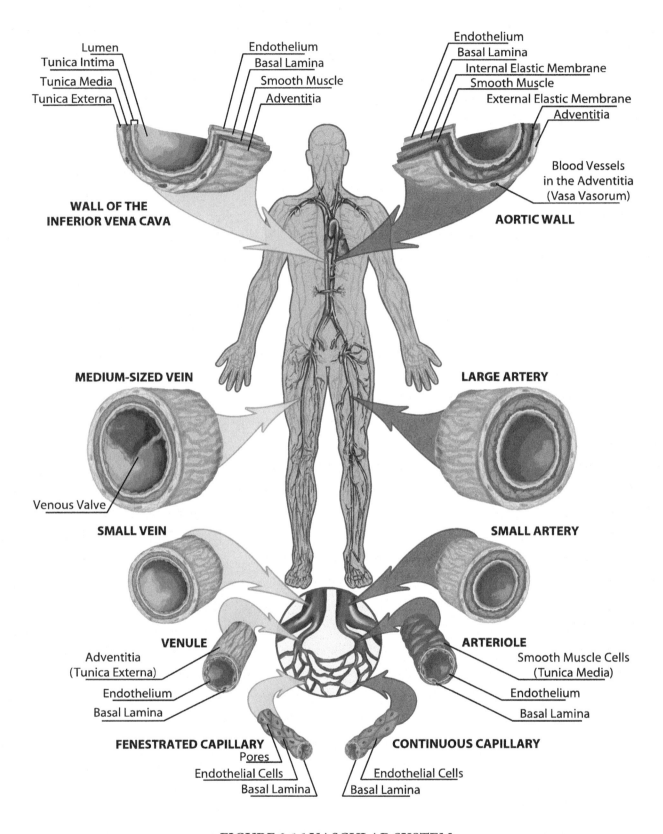

FIGURE 2.16 VASCULAR SYSTEM

VEINS FOR PHLEBOTOMY

Dorsal Metacarpal Vein

Cephalic Vein

Basilic Vein

Median Cubital Vein

Antecubital fossa

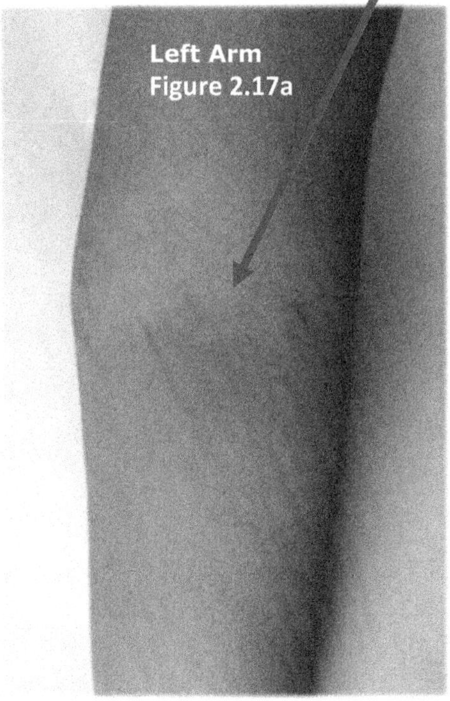

Left Arm
Figure 2.17a

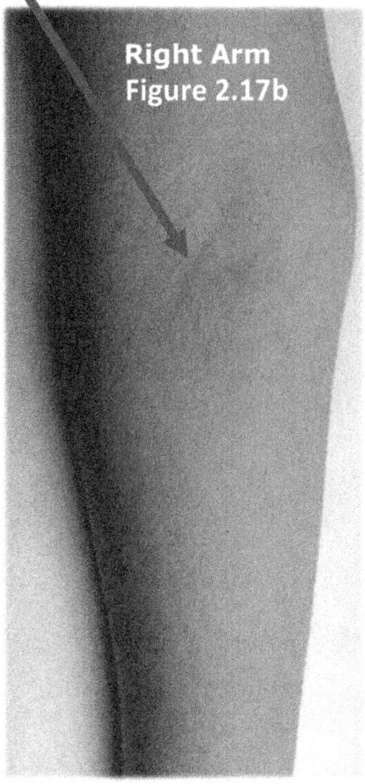

Right Arm
Figure 2.17b

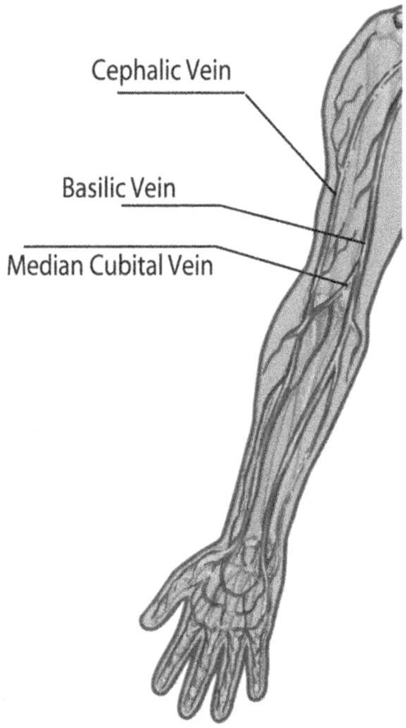

Cephalic Vein

Basilic Vein

Median Cubital Vein

Figure 2.18

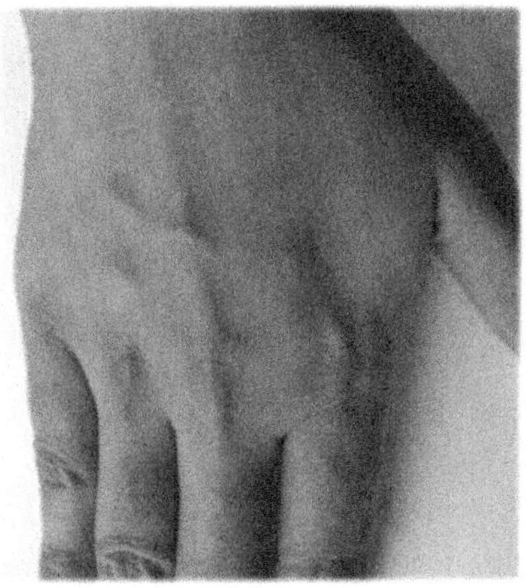

Right Hand
Figure 2.19a

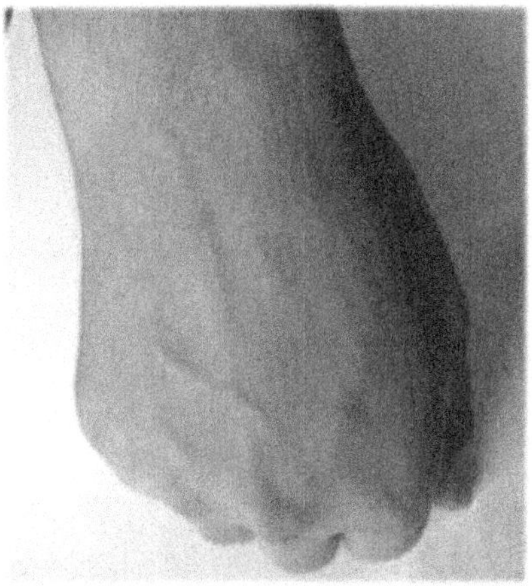

Right Hand (Clenched Fist)
Figure 2.19b

HUMAN ANATOMY: INTRODUCTION TO INTEGUMENTARY SYSTEM

The Integumentary system is an organ that includes skin, hair, nails, and sweat glands.

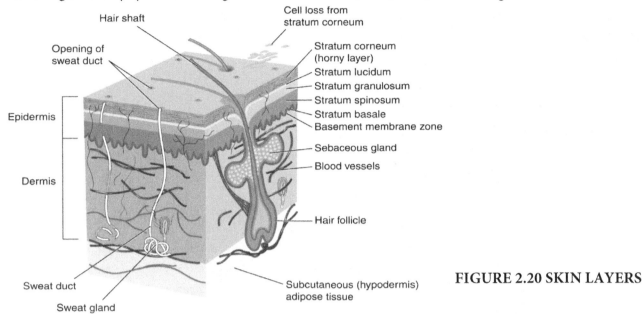

FIGURE 2.20 SKIN LAYERS

SKIN LAYERS

The human skin consists of 3 layer:
The three layers are as follows:

1. The innermost layer is called the **hypodermis** or **subcutaneous layer**.
2. The middle layer is called the **dermis**.
3. The outermost layer is called the **epidermis.**

LAYER	NAME
INNER	Hypodermis
	Dermis
MIDDLE	• Upper papillary layer
	• Lower reticular layer
	Epidermis
	(Upper to lower layers of epidermis)
	• Stratum Corneum
OUTER	• Stratum Lucidum
	• Stratum Granulosum
	• Stratum Spinosum
	• Stratum Basale

INNERMOST LAYER: HYPODERMIS/SUBCUTANEOUS LAYER

The innermost layer of the skin, hypodermis or the subcutaneous layer is composed of fat cells known as the adipocytes. The adipocytes are cells that stores fat. This storage of fat also functions as an energy reserve and is utilized when required. This layer by storing fat functions to insulate the body from external temperature. On the other hand, this layer also helps protect the body by absorbing shocks from outside the body on the skin.

MIDDLE LAYER: DERMIS

The dermis is the middle layer of the skin. It is situated between the below hypodermis and above epidermis.

THE DERMIS CONSISTS OF THE FOLLOWING LAYERS:

• UPPER PAPILLARY LAYER
• LOWER RETICULAR LAYER

OUTERMOST LAYER: EPIDERMIS

The epidermis is the outermost layer of the skin. This layer consists of the following layers.

• Stratum Corneum
• Stratum Lucidum
• Stratum Granulosum
• Stratum Spinosum
• Stratum Basale

The pathway of blood flow through the heart

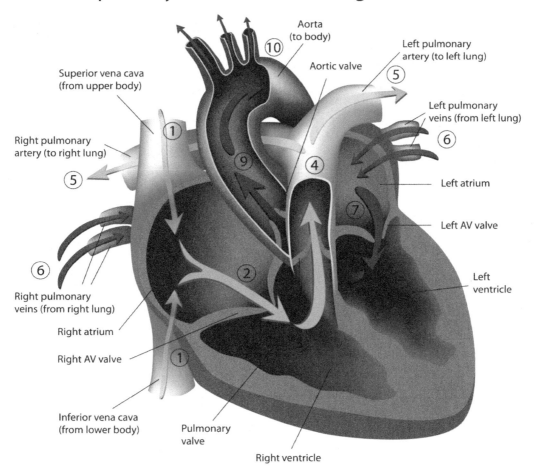

FIGURE 2.21 ANATOMY OF HEART

	RIGHT	**LEFT**
UPPER CHAMBERS	**ATRIUM** Receives deoxygenated blood from superior and inferior vena cava.	**ATRIUM** Receives oxygenated blood from both (right and left) lungs via the pulmonary vein.
LOWER CHAMBERS	**VENTRICLE** Receives the deoxygenated blood from right atrium via the tricuspid valve and pumps it out of the heart via the pulmonary artery to the right and the left lung.	**VENTRICLE** Receives oxygenated blood from left atrium via the bicuspid valve and pumps it out of the heart to the rest of the body via the aorta.

Table 2.5 HEART: INTERNAL BLOOD FLOW

HUMAN ANATOMY: INTRODUCTION TO PULMONARY SYSTEM

The respiratory system also known as the pulmonary system is the system of the human body. The main function of the respiratory system occurs through the process of inspiration and expiration. Inspiration is also known as inhalation, a process through which oxygen is inhaled into the lungs through the nose. Expiration is also known as exhalation, a process through which carbon-dioxide is exhaled out of the lungs through the nose. The process of inspiration and expiration combined can be referred to as the respiration. Organs, tissues, and cells in the human body require oxygen for proper functioning. On the other hand, the organs, tissues, and cells in the human body also need the removal of the carbon dioxide from the organs, tissues, and cells for proper functioning. This exchange of oxygen and carbon dioxide occurs continuously with the help of respiratory system.

The respiratory system is composed of two parts:
1. Upper Respiratory System
2. Lower Respiratory System

Upper Respiratory System
• Nose
• Nasal cavity
• Sinuses
• Pharynx
• Larynx

Lower Respiratory System
• Trachea
• Lungs
o Bronchi
o Bronchioles
o Alveoli

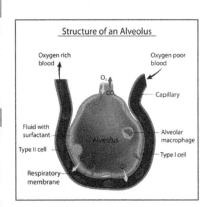

THE PROCESS OF RESPIRATION

It starts with the person inhaling air. The air inhaled through the nose passes into the pharynx, next passes into the larynx. After larynx, the air travels into the trachea and enter the lungs (right lung and left lung). Once the air inhaled enter the lungs, it passes through the bronchi, further to bronchioles and finally to the alveoli. At the alveolar level is where the gaseous exchange takes place. The gaseous exchange occurs by the oxygen entering the

capillary bloodstream from the alveoli and carbon dioxide exiting the capillary bloodstream into the alveoli. The oxygen collected by the capillary is supplied to the body and carbon dioxide collected by the alveoli is expelled out of the human body by the process of exhalation.

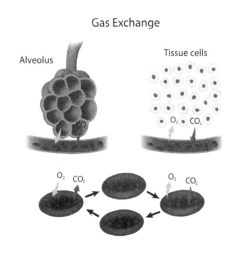

FIGURE 2.22 Gas Exchange at alveolar level

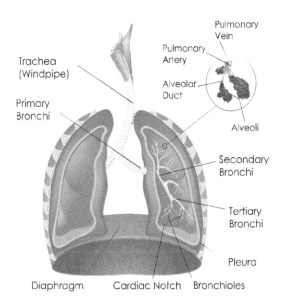

FIGURE 2.23 Pulmonary System

HUMAN ANATOMY: INTRODUCTION TO SKELETON SYSTEM

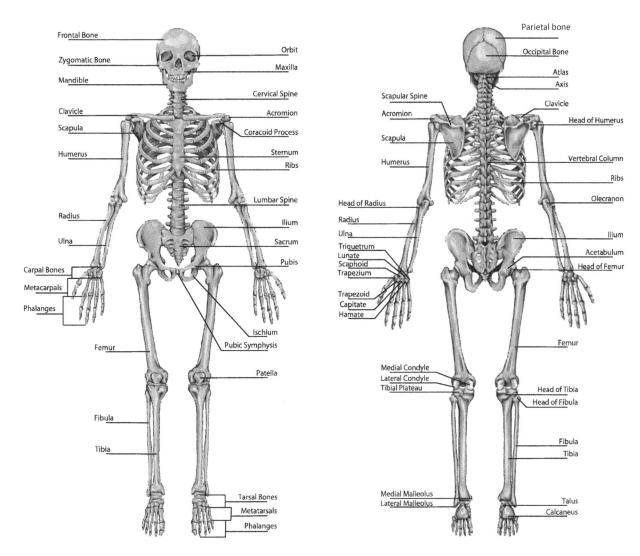

FIGURE 2.24 SKELETON SYSTEM FRONT VIEW (ANTERIOR) & BACK VIEW (POSTERIOR)

SKELETON SYSTEM IS DIVIDED INTO TWO SECTIONS

AXIAL SKELETON

A. SKULL
B. SPINAL COLUMN
C. SACRUM
D. RIBS
E. STERNUM

APPENDICULAR SKELETON

A. SHOULDER GIRDLE:
- CLAVICLE
- SCAPULA

B. PELVIC GIRDLE:
- PELVIS

C. ARM & HAND:
- HUMERUS
- ULNA
- RADIUS
- CARPALS
- METACARPALS
- PHALANGES

D. LEG AND FOOT:
- FEMUR
- PATELLA
- TIBIA
- FIBULA
- TARSALS
- METATARSALS
- PHALANGES

HUMAN ANATOMY: INTRODUCTION TO NERVOUS SYSTEM

Nervous system is made up of two parts:

a)   Central Nervous System (CNS) -brain and spinal cord

b)   Peripheral Nervous System (PNS) -motor neurons and sensory neurons

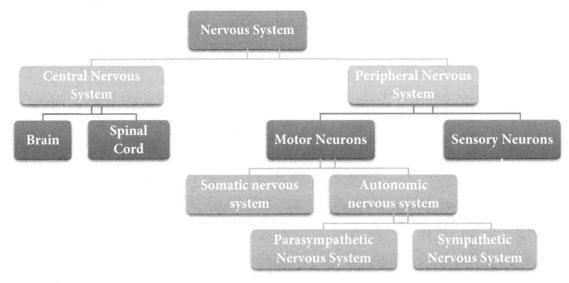

FIGURE 2.25 NERVOUS SYSTEM DIVISIONS

THE CENTRAL NERVOUS SYSTEM (CNS)

Is a part of the nervous system. It consists of two main components:

1. **The spinal cord**
    *   Carry and transfer signals between the brain and the rest of the body.
2. **The brain**
    *   Brain is located in the skull. The brain continues as the spinal cord in the vertebral canal.

THE PERIPHERAL NERVOUS SYSTEM (PNS)

Subdivided into the:

1) **Motor**
    A. Is further separated into somatic and autonomic nervous system:
        *   Somatic: Controls voluntary movement to muscles.
        *   Autonomic: Controls involuntary movement to muscles (smooth muscles, cardiac muscles, glands and adipose tissues). It is further separated into:
            i.   Sympathetic nervous system: Excitatory
            ii. Parasympathetic nervous system: Inhibitory

2) **Sensory**
    *   Sensory neuron brings information back to the Central Nervous System from the stimulus receiving receptor. For example: A person touching an ice cube will feel a sensation of cold on his or her skin, this occurs by the sensory neurons relaying information to the Central Nervous System. Similar to this other sensations are smell, hearing, vision, taste, balancing, etc.

HUMAN ANATOMY: INTRODUCTION TO URINARY SYSTEM

KIDNEYS

Kidneys are present in a pair, two in number. They play a vital role in the urinary system. All major processes of the urinary system occur in the kidneys. They are present in the back (abdominal region) and are bean shaped.

URETERS

Ureters are tubes that carry urine from the kidney to the urinary bladder. The ureters are two in number, namely the right ureter from the right kidney and the left ureter from the left kidney.

URINARY BLADDER

Urinary blabber is a bag or sac that is located in the lower abdominal region. The main function of the bladder is to hold the urine until it is expelled out via the urethra. The process of urination is often known as micturition.

URETHRA

The urethra is the structure through which the urine is expelled out of the urinary bladder. It serves as a passage for passing the urine from (out of the) the bladder to the out of the human body. The size of the male and female urethra are different. In general, Male urethra is longer than the female urethra.

NEPHRON

The Nephrons are the structural working units of the kidney. Their function is that of a filter. Blood entering the nephron is filtered, the end result being that majority of the constituents and water

is retained by the body, while the rest are excreted out of the kidney into the ureter.

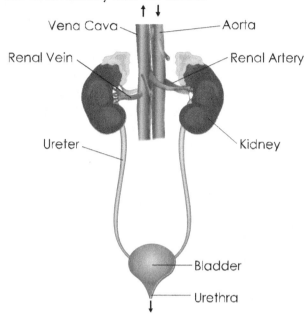

FIGURE 2.26 PARTS OF URINARY SYSTEM

EXCRETION OF URINE

The passage of urine out of the human body is known as urination. Other term used are micturition. This simply means, voiding the urine. The process of urination usually occurs when the bladder is full with urine, when this occurs, a sensory impulse is sent to the central nervous system (CNS) informing the CNS that the bladder is full with urine, receiving the information, the CNS through the motor nervous system causes the bladder to contract and sphincter muscles to relax. This contraction of the bladder and relaxation of the sphincter muscles results in voiding of the urine out of the human body.

HUMAN ANATOMY: INTRODUCTION TO DIGESTIVE SYSTEM

MOUTH

The mouth is the first part of the digestive system. It is the part where the digestive system starts. Mouth functions to intake food and break the food down into small parts before it is further passed into the digestive system. The food present in the mouth mixes with saliva and is broken down into small parts by chewing the food with the help of teeth's. Another structure present within the mouth is the tongue. The tongue helps in moving the food to either side of the mouth to be chewed. Another structure present is the salivary glands that causes the release of saliva that is mixed with food before and while it is being chewed.

ESOPHAGUS

Food from the mouth after being chewed is further passed into the esophagus. The esophagus is a tube-like structure that passes the food from the mouth into the bag like structure known as the stomach. The process of food passage through the esophagus occurs by peristalsis.

STOMACH

After receiving the chewed food from the mouth through the esophagus, the food enters the stomach. The food is further broken down by mixing of the food and gastric fluids of the stomach. This causes the food to be broken down further for easy digestion. The chewed food at this stage is known as **chyme**.

INTESTINES

The food from the stomach is further passed into the parts of the small intestine. The small intestine consists of the duodenum, jejunum and the ileum. The small intestine functions to absorb the constituents required by the human body, while the rest is further passed onto the large intestine where the water from the waste matter is reabsorbed. The large intestine consist of Cecum, Colon (Ascending colon, Transverse colon, Descending colon, Sigmoid colon) and the Rectum. The process of passing waste material out of the body through the rectum is referred to as **defecation**.

LIVER

Large gland that has two major portions namely the right and left. Liver produces bile. The main function of the bile is to break fat into smaller particles for better absorption. The liver also plays an important role in metabolism, detoxification, storage, and immunity.

GALLBLADDER

The location of the gallbladder is under the liver. The main function of the gall bladder is to release the stored bile into the small intestine mainly the duodenum when food containing fat is found. The bile causes the fat to be broken down into small particles for easy absorption.

PANCREAS

The pancreas plays a vital role in the process of digestive and regulation of blood sugar levels. It is both an endocrine gland and an exocrine gland. The endocrine function of the pancreas is that of the two hormones that it releases, insulin and glucagon. Insulin is released by the pancreas when the blood sugar level is in high concentration. On the other hand, glucagon is released by the pancreas when the blood sugar level is in low concentration.

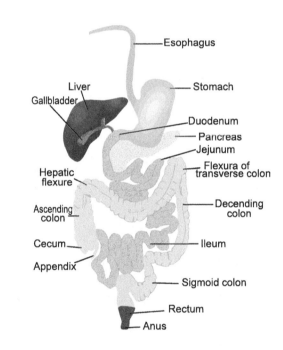

Fig 2.27 STAGES OF SWALLOWING

HUMAN ANATOMY: INTRODUCTION TO ENDOCRINE SYSTEM

The human body has various glands. Endocrine glands are the glands in the human body that release hormones. Hormones secreted by the glands are released into the blood stream. The hormones released; travel through the blood stream to reach its target organ where it is required. There are several endocrine glands in the human body and their respective hormones they release.

GLANDS OF THE HUMAN BODY

Glands	Hormones
ADRENAL GLANDS	• **Cortisol** • **Aldosterone** • **Epinephrine** • **Norepinephrine**
HYPOTHALAMUS	Secretes several releasing hormones: • **Thyrotropin-releasing hormone** • **Corticotropin-releasing hormone**
OVARIES	• **Estrogen** • **Progesterone**
PITUITARY GLAND This gland has two lobes: Anterior and Posterior	**Anterior Pituitary** • Growth hormone • Thyroid-stimulating hormone • Follicle-stimulating hormone • Luteinizing hormone • Prolactin • Adrenocorticotropic hormone • Melanocyte-stimulating hormone. **Posterior Pituitary** • Antidiuretic • Oxytocin

PARATHYROID	• **Parathyroid hormone (PTH)**
PANCREAS	• **Insulin** • **Glucagon**
THYROID GLAND	• **Triiodothyronine (T3)** • **Thyroxine (T4)**
THYMUS	• **Thymus hormones**
TESTES	• **Testosterone**

Table 2.6

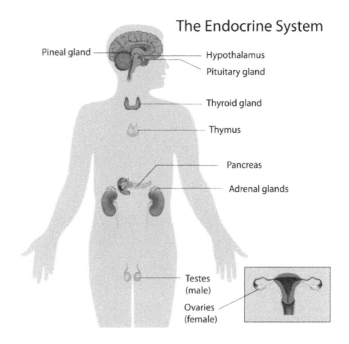

FIGURE 2.28 ENDOCRINE GLANDS

BODY PLANES

Coronal Plane or Frontal Plane – divides the human body into front and back.

Sagittal Plane or Median Plane – divides the human body into left & right.

Transverse Plane or Horizontal Plane – divides the human body into upper and lower parts.

DIRECTIONAL TERMS

Ventral/Anterior – Front of the body.

Dorsal/Posterior – Back of the body.

Lateral – Towards the side

Medial – Towards the center of the body.

Distal – Away from a point of reference

Proximal – Towards a point of reference

Superior – On top

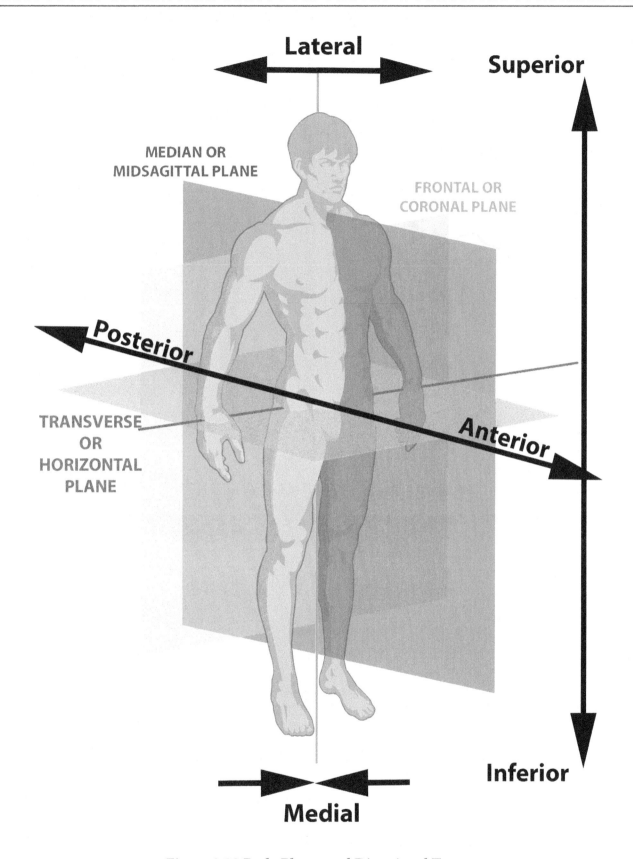

Figure 2.29 Body Planes and Directional Terms

ANATOMICAL MOVEMENTS

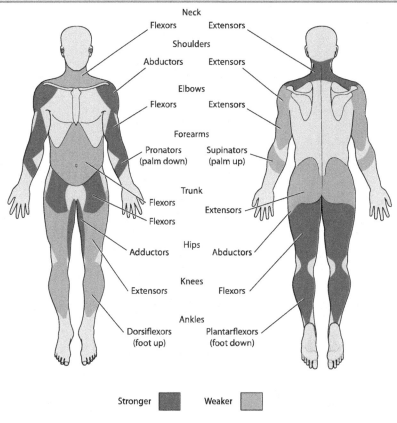

FIGURE 2.30 ANATOMICAL MOVEMENTS

MOVEMENT TERMINOLOGIES	
TERMS	**MEANING**
Flexion	Bones coming together or when the joint angle decreases.
Extension	When joint angle increases.
Abduction	Movement away from the midline of the body.
Adduction	Movement towards the midline of the body.
Internal rotation	Inward rotation, towards the midline of the body.
External rotation	Outward rotation, away from the midline of the body.
Circumduction	Combination of all the movements.
Pronation	Elbow at mid flexed position and palm facing downwards.
Supination	Elbow at mid flexed position and palm facing upwards.
Dorsi-flexion	Ankle joint flexes towards the leg (shin bone) or toes pointing towards the leg.
Plantar-flexion	Opposite of dorsiflexion.
Inversion	Turning of the ankle joint inward.
Eversion	Turning of the ankle joint outward.

Table 2.7

CHAPTER 2
END OF CHAPTER REVIEW QUESTIONS

Question Set 1: MATCH THE FOLLOWING

Answers	Column A	Column B
	Vasodilation	A. divides the body into front and back
	Ventral	B. back of the body
	Coronal Plane or Frontal plane	C. widening of blood vessels
	Sagittal plane or Median Plane.	D. furthest from the point
	Transverse plane or Horizontal Plane	E. front of the body
	Dorsal	F. narrowing of blood vessels
	Medial	G. divides the body into left & right
	Distal	H. towards the center of the body
	Vasoconstriction	I. closest to the point
	Proximal	J. divides the body into upper and lower parts

Question Set 2: ESSAY QUESTIONS

1. Explain the pulmonary system.
2. Describe in detail the elements of blood.
3. Explain blood serum and blood plasma.
4. Explain the process of hemostasis.
5. In brief, explain the human skeleton system.
6. Explain the different types of blood vessels in the human body.
7. Name and explain the layers of the skin.
8. In brief, explain the urinary and digestive system?
9. In brief, explain the endocrine system and list atleast 10 hormones.
10. Compare and contrast arteries and veins.

Question Set 3: Fill in the blanks

1. Plasma makes up _____% of the blood.

2. Plasma is made of _____% water.

3. _____ make up the remaining 45% of the blood.

4. Red blood cells make up _____% of the blood cells.

5. _____ make up the approximate 1% of the formed elements.

6. The normal range in men of RBC's is approximately _____to _____million cells/µl (microliter). The normal range in women for RBC's ranges from _____to _____million cells/µl, according to NIH (National Institutes of Health) data.

7. Separating plasma from the blood can be done by obtaining blood in a blood collection tube, followed by centrifuging the tube for _____ minutes at recommended rotations per minutes in a centrifuge device.

8. If an individual has Rh antigen _____, the individual is Rh negative for that particular blood group. If an individual has Rh antigen _____, the individual is Rh positive for that particular blood group.

9. _____ is a process by which the cells called phagocytes ingest or engulf other cells or particles.

10. Separating serum from the blood can be done by obtaining blood in a blood collection tube, and letting the blood to clot for _____ minutes, followed by centrifuging the blood collection tube for _____ minutes at recommended rotations per minutes in a centrifuge device.

Question Set 4: Multiple Choice Questions

1. Blood is a type of connective tissue and is fluid in nature. Its main function is to carry
   _____a)   carbon dioxide from the lungs to the body and carry oxygen from the body to the lungs
   _____b)   oxygen from the veins to the body and carry carbon dioxide from the body to the lungs
   _____c)   oxygen from the lungs to the body and carry carbon dioxide from the body to the lungs
   _____d)   carbon mono-oxide from the lungs to the body and carry carbon dioxide from the body to the lungs

2. Which of the following is not a stage of hemostasis?
   _____a)   Vasoconstriction
   _____b)   Thrombus formation
   _____c)   Platelet plug formation
   _____d)   Coagulation of blood

3. Which of the following is not the Stages of Blood Clotting?
   _____a)   Formation of prothrombin activator
   _____b)   Conversion of thrombin into prothrombin
   _____c)   Conversion of prothrombin into thrombin
   _____d)   Conversion of fibrinogen to fibrin

4. Which of the following vein is not found in the upper limbs?
   _____a)   Dorsal Metacarpal Vein
   _____b)   Cephalic Vein
   _____c)   Popliteal Vein
   _____d)   Median Cubital Vein

5. Which of the following is not the layer of skin?
   _____a)   Dermis
   _____b)   Epidermis
   _____c)   Subcutaneous Fat
   _____d)   Collagen

6. The epidermis is the outermost layer of the skin. Which of the following are the horizontal layers of the epidermis.
   _____a)   1ST Layer: Stratum Basale
   _____b)   2ND Layer: Stratum Spinosum
   _____c)   3RD Layer: Stratum Granulosum
   _____d)   All of the above

CHAPTER 3: MEDICAL TERMINOLOGY

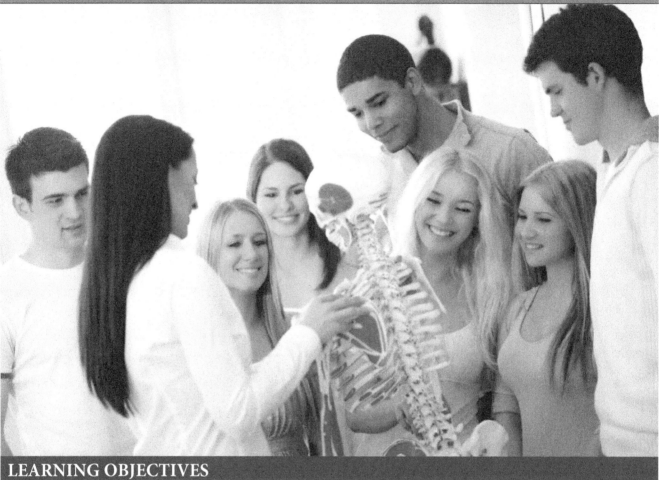

LEARNING OBJECTIVES

At the end of this chapter the student will be able to describe in brief:

- Part of the medical terminology.
- Common terms related to human body systems.
- Common medical terminologies.

EDICAL TERMINOLOGY

Medical terminology is the language that is used to describe the human body and associated components, conditions, disease, disorders, procedures and process.

Prefix

The prefix is the part of the medical terminology that may be added in front of the root word.

Suffix

The suffix is the part of the medical terminology that may be added to the end of the root word.

There are different parts of the medical terminology; let's discuss the parts:

ROOT	Gives meaning to the medical term
SUFFIX	This part is the one with which the medical term may end
PREFIX	This part is the one with which the medical term may start
COMBINING VOWEL	Is what combines a root to another root, a root to a suffix. (a, e, i, o, u)

Examples of Medical Terminology

Note:-The letters denotes   (R)= ROOT   (S)=SUFFIX   (P)= PREFIX   cv= combining vowel

CARDIOLOGY:	Cardi: heart (root)	O: (cv)		Logy: study of (suffix)
HEMATOLOGY:	Hemat: blood (root)	O: (cv)		Logy: study of (suffix)
NEUROLOGY:	Neuro: Brain (root)	O: (cv)		Logy: study of (suffix)
SUBGASTRIC:	Sub: below (prefix)		Gastr: stomach (root)	IC: pertaining to (suffix)

ummary:

Note the terms you will come across

Rules to follow

Never try to read it at one glance.

- *Break the term into parts.*
- *Understand each part of it.*
- *Join the words again.*
  - **Root:** gives the essential *meaning* of the term.
  - **Suffix:** is the word *ending*.
  - **Prefix:** is a small part added to the *beginning* of a term.
  - **Combining vowel:** connects roots to suffixes and roots to other roots.
  - **Combining form:** is the combination of the *root* and *combining vowel*.
- *Read* the meaning of the medical term from the suffix to the beginning of the word and then across.

Medical Terminology

A

Affix	Relating to	Suffix or Prefix	Word	Read
a or an	without	Prefix	**Anaerobic**	An-aero-bic
ab	away from	Prefix	**Abduction**	Ab-duc-tion
ad	towards	Prefix	**Adduction**	Ad-duc-tion
aden	gland	Prefix	**Adenocytes**	Adeno-cytes
adipo	fat	Prefix	**Adipose**	Adi-pose
adreno	adrenal glands	Prefix	**Adrenaline**	Adre-na-line
-al	related to	Suffix	**Axial**	Ax-ial
-algia	pain	Suffix, Prefix	**Arthralgia**	Ar-thral-gia
andro	male	Prefix	**Androgen**	An-dro-gen
angio	vessel	Prefix	**Angiogenesis**	Angio-gene-sis
ante	towards front	Prefix	**Anterior**	An-te-rior
anti	prevent, oppose or against	Prefix	**Antihistamine**	An-ti-his-ta-mine
arter	artery	Prefix	**Arteriosclerosis**	Ar-terio-scle-ro-sis
arthro	joints of the human body	Prefix	**Arthritis**	Ar-thri-tis
aspir	removal	Prefix	**Aspiration**	As-pi-ra-tion
audi	hearing or sound	Prefix	**Auditory**	Au-di-to-ry
auri	ear	Prefix	**Auricular**	Au-ri-cu-lar
axill	armpit	Prefix	**Axillary Nerve**	Axi-llary Nerve

B

Affix	Relating to	Suffix or Prefix	Word	Read
bacteri	bacteria	Prefix	Bactericides	Bac-teri-cides
baro	pressure	Prefix	Barometer	Baro-me-ter
brachi	arm	Prefix	Brachial Artery	Bra-chi-al Ar-te-ry
brady	slowing	Prefix	Bradycardia	Bra-dy-car-dia
bronchi	bronchus	Prefix	Bronchitis	Bron-chi-tis
bi	two	Prefix	Biceps	Bi-ceps
burs	bursae	Prefix	Bursitis	Bur-si-tis

C

Affix	Relating to	Suffix or Prefix	Word	Read
carcino	cancer	Prefix	Carcinogenic	Car-ci-no-genic
cardio	heart	Prefix	Cardiology	Car-dio-logy
-cardium	heart	Suffix	Epicardium	Epi-car-di-um
carp	carpal bones	Prefix	Carpals	Car-pals
-centesis	perforation	Suffix	Paracentesis	Para-cen-te-sis
-cephalic	head	Suffix	Hydrocephalic	Hy-dro-ce-pha-lic
cephalo	head	Prefix	Cephalic vein	Ce-pha-lic vein
chondro	cartilage	Prefix	Chondromalacia	Chon-dro-ma-la-cia
chol	bile	Prefix	Cholecystectomy	Cho-le-cys-tec-tomy
-cidal	killing in nature	Suffix	Bactericidal	Bac-teri-ci-dal
-clast	break into fragments	Suffix	Osteoclast	Os-teo-clast

contra	opposite or against	Prefix	**Contraindication**	Con-tra-in-di-ca-tion
costo	rib	Prefix	**Costal Cartilage**	Cos-tal Car-ti-lage
-constrict	narrowing	Suffix	**Vasoconstriction**	Va-so-cons-tric-tion
cryo	cold	Prefix	**Cryotherapy**	Cry-o-therapy
cutane	skin	Prefix	**Cutaneous**	Cu-ta-ne-ous
cyano	blue color	Prefix	**Cyanosis**	C-ya-no-sis
cysto	urinary bladder	Prefix	**Cystoscopy**	Cys-to-sco-py
-cytes	cell	Prefix, Suffix	**Osteocytes**	Os-te-o-cytes
cyto	cell	Prefix, Suffix	**Cytology**	Cy-to-lo-gy

D

Affix	Relating to	Suffix or Prefix	Word	Read
dent	teeth	Prefix	**Dental**	Den-tal
dermato	skin	Prefix	**Dermatologist**	Der-ma-to-lo-gist
dextr	right side	Prefix	**Dextrocardiac**	Dex-tro-car-diac
dia	throughout or complete	Prefix	**Diagnosis**	Di-ag-no-sis
-dipsia	thirst	Suffix	**Polydipsia**	Po-ly-dip-sia
dors	back or behind	Prefix	**Dorsal**	Dor-sal
-dynia	painful	Suffix	**Urodynia**	Uro-dy-nia
dys	difficult	Prefix	**Dysphagia**	Dys-pha-gia

E

Affix	Relating to	Suffix or Prefix	Word	Read
-eal	related to	Suffix	**Esophageal**	Eso-pha-geal

-ectomy	surgical removal of a body part	Suffix	**Hysterectomy**	Hys-te-rec-to-my
-emesis	vomit	Suffix	**Hyperemesis**	Hy-per-eme-sis
encephalo	brain	Prefix	**Encephalography**	En-ce-pha-lo-gra-phy
endo	internal	Prefix	**Endothelium**	En-do-the-li-um
entero/i	intestine	Prefix	**Enteritis**	En-te-ri-tis
epi	above or upon	Prefix	**Epidermis**	Epi-der-mis
erythr	red	Prefix	**Erythrocytes**	Ery-thro-cytes
esthesi	sensation	Suffix	**Anaesthesia**	An-aes-the-sia
ex	outer	Prefix	**Exoderm**	Ex-o-derm

F

Affix	Relating to	Suffix or Prefix	Word	Read
faci	face	Prefix	**Facial Nerve**	Fa-ci-al Nerve
fossa	hollow area	Prefix	**Fossa Ovalis**	Fo-ssa Ova-lis
fungi	fungus	Prefix	**Fungal Infection**	Fun-gal In-fec-tion

G

Affix	Relating to	Suffix or Prefix	Word	Read
gastr	stomach	Prefix	**Gastritis**	Gas-tri-tis
genu	knee	Prefix	**Genu Recurvatum**	Ge-nu Re-cur-va-tum
-gnosis	knowledge	Suffix	**Prognosis**	Prog-no-sis
gonio	angle	Prefix	**Goniometry**	Go-ni-o-met-ry
-gram	recording	Suffix	**Electrocardiogram**	Elec-tro-car-di-o-gram
-graph	generating the recording	Suffix	**Electrocardiograph**	Elec-tro-car-di-o-graph

| -graphy | recording process | Suffix | **Electrocardiography** | Elec-tro-car-di-o-graphy |
| **gynae** | female | Prefix | **Gynaecology** | Gy-na-e-co-lo-gy |

H

Affix	Relating to	Suffix or Prefix	Word	Read
hemat	blood	Prefix	**Hematology**	He-ma-to-lo-gy
hemo	blood	Prefix	**Hemoglobin**	He-mo-glo-bin
hemi	half	Prefix	**Hemiplegia**	He-mi-ple-gia
hepat	liver	Prefix	**Hepatocytes**	He-pa-to-cytes
herni	hernia	Prefix	**Herniorrhaphy**	Her-ni-o-rrha-phy
hetero	different	Prefix	**Heterogeneous**	He-te-ro-ge-ne-ous
histo	tissue	Prefix	**Histology**	His-to-lo-gy
hydro	water	Prefix	**Hydrophobic**	Hy-dro-pho-bic
hyper	extreme or beyond	Prefix	**Hypertension**	Hy-per-ten-sion
hypo	below or under	Prefix	**Hypotension**	Hy-po-ten-sion
hyster	uterus	Prefix	**Hysterectomy**	Hys-te-rec-tomy

I

Affix	Relating to	Suffix or Prefix	Word	Read
infra	beneath or below	Prefix	**Infraspinatus**	In-fra-spi-na-tus
inter	between	Prefix	**Intercostal**	In-ter-cos-tal
intra	within	Prefix	**Intramuscular**	In-tra-mus-cu-lar
immun	protection or immune	Prefix	**Immune System**	Immune System
ipsi	same	Prefix	**Ipsilateral**	Ip-si-la-te-ral

-ism	condition, disease, disorder	Suffix	Parkinsonism	Par-kin-son-ism
iso	same	Prefix	Isometric	Iso-met-ric
-itis	inflammation	Suffix	Osteoarthritis	Os-teo-ar-thri-tis

K

Affix	Relating to	Suffix or Prefix	Word	Read
kinesio	movement	Prefix	Kinesiology	Ki-ne-sio-logy

L

Affix	Relating to	Suffix or Prefix	Word	Read
lact	lactic or milk	Prefix	Lactose Intolerance	Lac-tose Intolerance
laparo	abdomen	Prefix	Laparotomy	La-pa-ro-tomy
leuko	white	Prefix	Leukocytes	Leu-ko-cytes
levo or laevo	left	Prefix	Levocardia	Le-vo-car-dia
lipo	fat	Prefix	Lipoma	Li-po-ma
-logy	study of	Suffix	Cardiology	Car-di-o-logy
-lysis	destruction	Suffix	Spondylolysis	Spon-dy-lo-ly-sis

M

Affix	Relating to	Suffix or Prefix	Word	Read
macr	large	Prefix	Macrophage	Mac-ro-phage
-malacia	abnormal softening	Suffix	Osteomalacia	Os-te-o-ma-la-cia
mammo	breast	Prefix	Mammogram	Ma-mmo-gram
-megaly	enlargement	Suffix	Cardiomegaly	Car-di-o-me-ga-ly
melano	black	Prefix	Melanocytes	Me-la-no-cy-tes

-metry	measure	Suffix	Telemetry	Te-le-me-try
micro	small	Prefix	Microorganisms	Mi-cro-orga-ni-sms
mono	one	Prefix	Monoplegia	Mo-no-ple-gia
morpho	shape or character	Prefix	Morphology	Mor-pho-logy
muscul	muscle	Prefix	Musculoskeletal System	Mus-cu-lo-ske-le-tal System
myo	muscle	Prefix	Myology	Myo-logy
myco	fungus	Prefix	Mycobacteriosis	My-co-bac-te-ri-o-sis

N

Affix	Relating to	Suffix or Prefix	Word	Read
naso	nose	Prefix	Nasopharynx	Na-so-pha-ry-nx
necro	death	Prefix	Necrosis	Ne-cro-sis
neo	new	Prefix	Neoplasm	Ne-o-pla-sm
nephro	kidney	Prefix	Nephrology	Ne-phro-logy
nerv	nerves	Prefix	Nerve	Ner-ve
neur	nervous system	Prefix	Neuritis	Neu-ri-tis
nocti	night	Prefix	Nocturnal	Noc-tur-nal

O

Affix	Relating to	Suffix or Prefix	Word	Read
ocul	eye	Prefix	Oculomotor Nerve	Ocu-lo-mo-tor Nerve
odyn	pain	Prefix	Odynophagia	O-dy-no-pha-gia
-oma	tumor	Suffix	Carcinoma	Car-ci-no-ma
onco	tumor	Prefix	Oncology	On-co-logy

ophthal	eye	Prefix	Ophthalmology	Oph-thal-mo-logy
opistho	behind	Prefix	Opisthotonic Posturing	Opis-tho-to-nic Posturing
-osis	condition, disease, disorder	Suffix	Osteoporosis	Os-te-o-po-ro-sis
osteo	bone	Prefix	Osteocytes	Os-te-o-cytes

P

Affix	Relating to	Suffix or Prefix	Word	Read
para	beside	Suffix	Parathyroid Gland	Pa-ra-thy-ro-id Gland
-paresis	weakness	Suffix	Hemiparesis	Hemi-pa-re-sis
patho	disease	Prefix	Pathology	Pa-tho-logy
-pathy	disorder	Suffix	Osteopathy	Os-te-o-pathy
pedo	child	Prefix	Pediatric	Pe-dia-tric
-penia	deficiency	Suffix	Leucopenia	Leu-co-pe-nia
per	through or completely	Prefix	Perforation	Per-fo-ra-tion
peri	surrounding or around	Prefix	Pericardium	Pe-ri-car-di-um
phagia	eating	Suffix	Dysphagia	Dys-pha-gia
-phasia	speech	Suffix	Aphasia	A-pha-sia
phleb	vein	Prefix	Phlebotomy	Phle-bo-to-my
-phobia	fear of	Suffix	Hydrophobia	Hy-dro-pho-bia
-physis	growth	Suffix	Osteophysis	Os-te-o-phy-sis
-plasm	develop	Suffix	Neoplasm	Ne-o-pla-sm
-plasty	reconstructive surgery	Suffix	Angioplasty	An-gio-pla-s-ty
-plegia	paralysis	Suffix	Hemiplegia	He-mi-ple-gia

pneumo	lungs	Prefix	**Pneumonia**	P-neu-mo-nia
-pnea	breathing	Suffix	**Apnea**	A-p-ne-a
post	after	Prefix	**Post-operative**	Post-operative
pre	before	Prefix	**Pre-operative**	Pre-operative
pulmo	lungs	Prefix	**Pulmonary**	Pul-mo-na-ry

R

Affix	Meaning	Suffix or Prefix	Word	Read
rhin	nose	Prefix	**Rhinoplasty**	Rhi-no-plas-ty
-rrhage	flow of discharge	Suffix	**Hemorrhage**	He-mo-rrha-ge
-rrhagia	abnormal flow of discharge	Suffix	**Hemorrhagia**	He-mo-rrha-gia
-rrhaphy	suture	Suffix	**Herniorrhaphy**	Her-ni-o-rrha-phy
-rrhea	discharge	Suffix	**Rhinorrhea**	Rhi-no-rrhea

S

Affix	Relating to	Suffix or Prefix	Word	Read
semi	half	Suffix	**Semipermeable**	Se-mi-per-me-a-ble
sero	serum	Suffix	**Serum**	Se-rum
-scope	examining instrument	Suffix	**Stethoscope**	Ste-tho-scope
-scopy	use of examining instrument	Suffix	**Arthroscopy**	Ar-thro-scopy
sinus	cavity	Prefix	**Sinusitis**	Si-nu-si-tis
somato	part of the body	Prefix	**Somatosensory**	So-ma-to-sen-so-ry
spondylo	vertebra	Prefix	**Spondylitis**	Spon-dy-li-tis
-stasis	slowing or stopping	Suffix	**Hemostasis**	He-mo-sta-sis

steno	narrowing	Prefix	Stenosis	Ste-no-sis
-stomy	a surgical procedure to create an opening.	Suffix	Ostomy	Os-to-my
sub	lower or under	Prefix	Sublingual	Sub-lin-gu-al
supra	above or over	Prefix	Supraspinatus Muscle	Su-pra-spi-natus Muscle

T

Affix	Relating to	Suffix or Prefix	Word	Read
tachy	fast	Prefix	Tachycardia	Ta-chy-car-dia
tele	distance	Prefix	Telemetry	Te-le-me-try
teno	tendon	Prefix	Tendinitis	Ten-di-ni-tis
tetra	four	Prefix	Tetraplegia	Te-tra-ple-gia
thorac	thorax or chest	Prefix	Thoracic Cavity	Tho-ra-cic Cavity
thrombo	blood clot	Prefix	Thrombosis	Thro-m-bo-sis
-tomy	surgical cut or incision	Suffix	Osteotomy	Os-teo-to-my
tox	toxin	Prefix, Suffix	Toxicology	To-xi-co-logy
trans	across	Prefix	Transplant	Trans-plant
tri	three	Prefix	Trimester	Tri-mes-ter
tympa	ear	Prefix	Tympanic Membrane	Tym-pa-nic Membrane

U

Affix	Relating to	Suffix or Prefix	Word	Read
uni	one	Prefix	Unipolar	Uni-po-lar
urina/o	urinary system	Prefix	Urinary System	Uri-na-ry System
uter	uterus (female)	Prefix	Uterus	Ute-rus

V

Affix	Relating to	Suffix or Prefix	Word	Read
vaso	vessel	Prefix	**Vasculitis**	Vas-cu-li-tis
ven	vein	Prefix	**Venipuncture**	Veni-punc-ture
vir	virus	Prefix	**Virology**	Vi-ro-lo-gy
viscero	organ	Prefix	**Visceral layer**	Vi-sce-ral layer
vitro	glass	Prefix	**Vitro fertilization**	Vi-tro fertilization

CHAPTER 3
END OF CHAPTER REVIEW QUESTIONS

Question Set 1: Fill in the Missing Answers

A

Affix	Relating to	Suffix or Prefix	Word
a or an	without		**Anaerobic**
ab	away from		**Abduction**
ad	towards		**Adduction**
aden	gland	Prefix	
adipo		Prefix	**Adipose**
adreno		Prefix	**Adrenaline**
-al		Suffix	**Axial**
-algia	pain	Suffix, Prefix	
andro		Prefix	**Androgen**

angio		Prefix	Angiogenesis
ante	towards front		Anterior
anti	prevent, oppose or against		Antihistamine
arter	artery	Prefix	
arthro		Prefix	Arthritis
aspiro	removal		Aspiration
audi		Prefix	Auditory
auri		Prefix	Auricular
axill	armpit	Prefix	

B

Affix	Relating to	Suffix or Prefix	Word
bacteri	bacteria		Bactericides
baro		Prefix	Barometer
brachi	arm	Prefix	
brady		Prefix	Bradycardia
bronchi	bronchus		Bronchitis
bi		Prefix	Biceps
burs	bursae	Prefix	

C

Affix	Relating to	Suffix or Prefix	Word
carcino	cancer		Carcinogenic
cardio		Prefix	Cardiology

-cardium	heart	Suffix	
carp		Prefix	**Carpals**
-centesis	perforation		**Paracentesis**
-cephalic	head	Suffix	
cephalo		Prefix	**Cephalic vein**
chondro	cartilage		**Chondromalacia**
chol	bile	Prefix	
-cidal		Suffix	**Bactericidal**
-clast	break into fragments		**Osteoclast**
contra	opposite or against	Prefix	
costo	.	Prefix	**Costal Cartilage**
-constrict	narrowing		**Vasoconstriction**
cryo	cold	Prefix	
cutane		Prefix	**Cutaneous**
cyano	blue color		**Cyanosis**
cysto	urinary bladder	Prefix	
-cytes		Prefix, Suffix	**Osteocytes**
cyto	cell	Prefix, Suffix	

D

Affix	Relating to	Suffix or Prefix	Word
dent	teeth	Prefix	
dermato		Prefix	**Dermatologist**

dextr	right side	Prefix	
dia	throughout or complete		Diagnosis
-dipsia	thirst	Suffix	
dors		Prefix	Dorsal
-dynia	painful		Urodynia
dys	difficult	Prefix	

E

Affix	Relating to	Suffix or Prefix	Word
-eal	related to	Suffix	Esophageal
-ectomy		Suffix	Hysterectomy
-emesis	vomit	Suffix	
encephalo		Prefix	Encephalography
endo		Prefix	Endothelium
entero/i		Prefix	Enteritis
epi		Prefix	Epidermis
erythr		Prefix	Erythrocytes
esthesi		Suffix	Anaesthesia
ex		Prefix	Exoderm

F

Affix	Relating to	Word
faci		Facial Nerve
fossa		Fossa Ovalis

fungi		Fungal Infection

G

Affix	Relating to	Word
gastr		Gastritis
genu		Genu Recurvatum
-gnosis		Prognosis
gonio		Goniometry
-gram		Electrocardiogram
-graph		Electrocardiograph
-graphy		Electrocardiography
gynae		Gynaecology

H

Affix	Relating to	Word
hemat		Hematology
hemo		Hemoglobin
hemi		Hemiplegia
hepat		Hepatocytes
herni		Herniorrhaphy
hetero		Heterogeneous
histo		Histology
hydro		Hydrophobic
hyper		Hypertension

hypo		Hypotension
hyster		Hysterectomy

I

Affix	Relating to	Word
infra		Infraspinatus
inter		Intercostal
intra		Intramuscular
immun		Immune System
ipsi		Ipsilateral
-ism		Parkinsonism
iso		Isometric
-itis		Osteoarthritis

K

Affix	Relating to	Word
kinesio		Kinesiology

L

Affix	Relating to	Word
lact		Lactose Intolerance
laparo		Laparotomy
leuko		Leukocytes
levo or laevo		Levocardia
lipo		Lipoma

-logy		Cardiology
-lysis		Spondylolysis

M

Affix	Relating to	Word
macr		Macrophage
-malacia		Osteomalacia
mammo		Mammogram
-megaly		Cardiomegaly
melano		Melanocytes
-metry		Telemetry
micro		Microorganisms
mono		Monoplegia
morpho		Morphology
muscul		Musculoskeletal System
myo		Myology
myco		Mycobacteriosis

N

Affix	Relating to	Word
naso		Nasopharynx
necro		Necrosis
neo		Neoplasm
nephro		Nephrology

nerv		Nerve
neur		Neuritis
nocti		Nocturnal

O

Affix	Relating to	Word
ocul		Oculomotor Nerve
odyn		Odynophagia
-oma		Carcinoma
onco		Oncology
ophthal		Ophthalmology
opistho		Opisthotonic Posturing
-osis		Osteoporosis
osteo		Osteocytes

P

Affix	Relating to	Word
para		Parathyroid Gland
-paresis		Hemiparesis
patho		Pathology
-pathy		Osteopathy
pedo		Pediatric
-penia		Leucopenia
per		Perforation

peri		Pericardium
phagia		Dysphagia
-phasia		Aphasia
phleb		Phlebotomy
-phobia		Hydrophobia
-physis		Osteophysis
-plasm		Neoplasm
-plasty		Angioplasty
-plegia		Hemiplegia
pneumo		Pneumonia
-pnea		Apnea
post		Post-operative
pre		Pre-operative
pulmo		Pulmonary

R

Affix	Meaning	Word
rhin		Rhinoplasty
-rrhage		Hemorrhage
-rrhagia		Hemorrhagia
-rrhaphy		Herniorrhaphy
-rrhea		Rhinorrhea

S

Affix	Relating to	Word
semi		Semipermeable
sero		Serum
-scope		Stethoscope
-scopy		Arthroscopy
sinus		Sinusitis
somato		Somatosensory
spondylo		Spondylitis
-stasis		Hemostasis
steno		Stenosis
-stomy		Ostomy
sub		Sublingual
supra		Supraspinatus Muscle

T

Affix	Relating to	Word
tachy		Tachycardia
tele		Telemetry
teno		Tendinitis
tetra		Tetraplegia
thorac		Thoracic Cavity
thrombo		Thrombosis

-tomy		Osteotomy
tox		Toxicology
trans		Transplant
tri		Trimester
tympa		Tympanic Membrane

U

Affix	Relating to	Word
uni		Unipolar
urina/o		Urinary System
uter		Uterus

V

Affix	Relating to	Word
vaso		Vasculitis
ven		Venipuncture
vir		Virology
viscero		Visceral layer
vitro		Vitro fertilization

EQUIPMENT & SUPPLIES

CHAPTER 4: PHLEBOTOMY EQUIPMENT & SUPPLIES

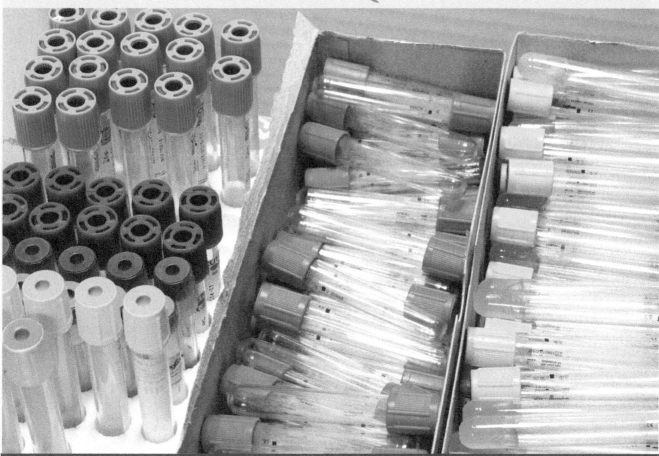

LEARNING OBJECTIVES

At the end of this chapter the student will be able to describe in brief:

Gloves

Tourniquet

Alcohol pads

Gauze

Bandage

Needles

Needle holder

Sharps container

Evacuated blood collection tubes & tube inversion technique

Blood specimens in phlebotomy

Tube additives

Blood collection color coded tube

Order of draw

Dermal puncture

Understanding capillary blood

Equipment & supplies required for dermal puncture

    Containers

    Capillary tubes

    Lancet

    Warming device

Dermal puncture order of draw

Centrifuge

Specimen processing

PHLEBOTOMY EQUIPMENT & SUPPLIES

Equipment & supplies needed includes needles, tubes, sharps disposal container, needle holders, syringes, winged infusion sets, gloves, tourniquets, antiseptic, gauze, and bandages.

The phlebotomy technician must be familiar with the equipment and supplies that are required to perform the phlebotomy procedure. The phlebotomy technician must correctly identify and gather equipment that will be required to perform the procedure. The equipment is usually gathered in a phlebotomy tray or cart. The equipment and supplies that will be gathered for the procedure must be checked for their expiration date and manufacturing defects. In this chapter, we will learn about the commonly used equipment and supplies that are required to performed the venipuncture procedure.

Inpatient vs. Out Patient

- If the patient is admitted to the hospital, the phlebotomy technician will be required to locate the patient and visit the patient's room to draw blood.
- If the patient is in a medical office, the patient may be required to visit the lab area or a room designated for drawing blood. However, this varies from facility to facility.

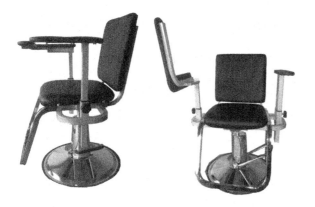

Figure 4.1 Phlebotomy Chair

Equipment and supplies required for each technique:

Venipuncture using a Multisample Needle Method

1. Needle (with or without safety lock)
2. Tube Holder
3. Tube
4. Alcohol Pad
5. Cotton
6. Gauze
7. Bandage
8. Sharps container
9. Gloves
10. Tourniquet

Venipuncture using a Winged Infusion Needle Method

1. Butterfly Needle
2. Tube Holder
3. Tube
4. Alcohol Pad
5. Cotton
6. Gauze
7. Bandage
8. Sharps container
9. Gloves
10. Tourniquet

Venipuncture using a Syringe Method

1. Syringe & Needle
2. Transfer Device
3. Tube
4. Alcohol Pad
5. Cotton
6. Gauze
7. Bandage
8. Sharps container
9. Gloves
10. Tourniquet

Glucose Testing

1. Lancet
2. Alcohol Pad
3. Cotton
4. Gauze or Bandage
5. Sharps container

6. Gloves
7. Glucose Test Strip
8. Glucose Analyzer Machine

Capillary Test

1. Lancet
2. Capillary Tube
3. Alcohol Pad
4. Cotton
5. Gauze or Bandage
6. Sharps container
7. Gloves
8. Hematocrit centrifuge
9. Clay sealant

Bleeding Time Test

1. Lancet
2. Alcohol Pad
3. Cotton
4. Gauze or Bandage
5. Sharps container
6. Gloves
7. Blood Pressure Set
8. Timer
9. Filter Paper

GLOVES

Mainly of two types

✓ **Sterile**: used for sterile procedure like surgeries
✓ **Non-Sterile**: used for phlebotomy

Gloves are available in different Sizes, Colors, and Materials

✓ Sizes: (e.g. Small, Medium, and Large)
✓ Colors: White, Blue, Lavender, and Green
✓ Materials: Latex, Non-Latex, Synthetic Vinyl, and Nitrile

Steps in wearing gloves:

1. Perform hand hygiene.
2. Select proper size gloves.
3. Don (wear) gloves.
4. Perform the procedure.

Steps in removing gloves:

1. Post-procedure.
2. Remove gloves.

3. Discard them into their appropriate container.
4. Perform hand hygiene.

Most of the medical facilities use non-latex gloves, since patients may be allergic to latex. Also, the powder on the latex gloves may contaminate the specimen. Gloves once used must not be reused on another patient, since doing so increase the chances of cross infection.

Gloves should be removed and discarded if

1. They are soiled with blood,
2. After contact with patient,
3. If they are damaged or torn.

Glove selection by the phlebotomy technician.

The phlebotomy technician must select the most appropriate sized glove that he or she may use for the procedure.

- If the glove is too large, the phlebotomy technician may have difficulty holding the equipment and supplies properly making it difficult to perform the procedure.
- If the gloves are too small, it may tightly fit on the hand and thereby restrict the hand movements, making it difficult to perform the procedure.

Hence, the correct size gloves must be chosen to perform the procedure.

TOURNIQUET

Tourniquet is an elastic band like strip that is wrapped or tied around the patient's arm. The main function of the tourniquet is to create pressure and make the vein prominent or visible for venipuncture. The tourniquet is available in standard sizes to suit the size of the patient's arm. They are made up of non-latex material and are elastic in nature, which means that it can be stretched to its yield point. They also come in a non-slip texture form so that it does not roll or slip on the skin.

Five points to consider when using tourniquet:

1. **The correct location should be selected prior to applying the tourniquet for performing the procedure.**
   - When performing venipuncture procedure on the arm (antecubital region), it is recommended that the tourniquet is applied **3-4 inches above the site of the puncture.**

2. **Appropriate pressure must be created while the tourniquet is in place.**

- The tourniquet should not be too tight on the patient's arm, since this may stop the flow of blood to the arm.
- The tourniquet should not be too loose on the patient's arm, since this may not create enough pressure required for the vein to become prominent.

3. **The tourniquet must be in place for recommended duration.**
    - The tourniquet once placed on the patient's arm must be untied/removed within **60 seconds or 1 minute**. It should not stay in place for more than **60 seconds or 1 minute**.

4. **Proper application and removal technique.**
    - The application must be such that it should not cause discomfort to the patient by either the application of the tourniquet being too tight or the tourniquet rolling up and pinching the skin.
    - The removal of the tourniquet must also be properly performed by untying (gently pull to release) one end of the tourniquet.

5. **Disposal of the tourniquet.**
    - The tourniquet must be disposed into their appropriate container after its use. It must not be reused onto another patient to avoid cross infection.

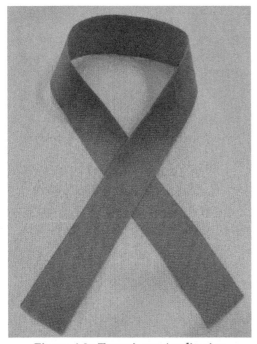

Figure 4.2a Tourniquet Application

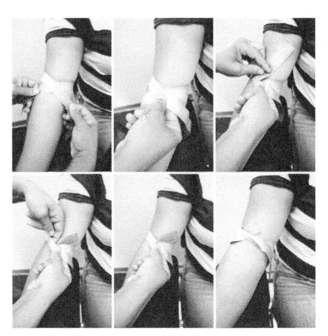

Figure 4.2b Tourniquet Application

ALCOHOL PADS

The most common topical antiseptic used in phlebotomy procedures is the 70% isopropyl alcohol pads. The alcohol pad is mainly used to clean and disinfect the site of the puncture. The pad consists of 70% isopropyl alcohol and 30% water. The 70% isopropyl alcohol is also referred to as the "rubbing alcohol" and "Alcohol Prep Pads". The pad is made up of cloth and has an alcohol odor to it. 70% rubbing isopropyl alcohol is unsafe for human consumption. In some cases skin irritation may occur when the isopropyl alcohol comes in contact with the patient's skin, if this occurs, it is usually recommended to discontinue its use on the patient. If it comes in contact with the eye, the eye should be rinsed with cool water.

Points to consider when using alcohol prep pads:

1. Cleaning and disinfecting the alcohol site must be done properly in concentric circles, moving from inside to outside or as recommended by the facility.
2. Post application of the topical alcohol prep pad on the surface of the skin, **let the skin air dry** before performing the procedure.
3. Check the **expiration date** of the product.
4. The alcohol prep pads come in an individually sealed alcohol prep packet, prior to opening the packet ensure that
    a. the **package is not damaged** or

b. the **seal is not opened.**

Alternative antiseptics used are

1. **Chlorhexidine gluconate** applicator, pad or swab.
2. **Iodine** applicator, pad or swab.
3. **Benzalkonium chloride** solution, pad or swab stick.

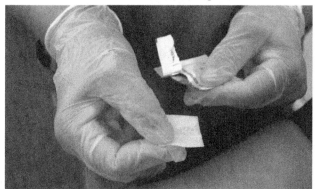

Figure 4.3 Alcohol Pads

GAUZE

Gauze is white in color and is usually odorless. It is available in various sizes depending on its use. The gauze that is used for phlebotomy procedures are **the clean 2×2 gauze pads.** A gauze pad is placed on the puncture site after the needle is withdrawn from the puncture site. Once the clean 2x2 gauze pad is in place, either the phlebotomy technician or the patient holding the gauze pad in place must ensure that appropriate pressure is being applied to the puncture site using the gauze pad. The pressure applied to the puncture site is to stop the puncture site from bleeding. After the bleeding has stopped, an adhesive bandage is applied to the site, and the 2x2 gauze pad is disposed into its appropriate container.

BANDAGE

Bandages are adhesive strips that are applied to the puncture site. The reason for applying the bandage on the puncture site is to:

1. Protect the area from direct exposure.
2. Assist in wound healing process

The parts of the bandage are:

1. Two side strips: The two side strips are adhesive in nature, and they adhere to the skin surface, once in contact with the skin.
2. One center pad: The center pad is of various types, they are usually absorbent in nature and may have an antiseptic on them.

While applying the bandage on the site after the phlebotomy procedure. Ensure that the center pad is the area of the bandage that is in contact with the puncture site since the puncture site is the site that requires protection from contamination. The correct technique must be practiced to apply bandage onto the puncture site as the application of bandage may not be easy, especially when the phlebotomy technician is applying the bandage with their gloves on. Some patients might be allergic to the bandage strip, in such patients use the self-adhesive gauze pads.

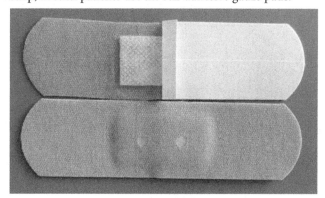

Figure 4.4 Bandage

NEEDLES

Needles are most commonly used equipment when drawing blood from the arm or hand region. Its function is to puncture the skin and enter the vein. Needles are available in different:

- Gauges
- Lengths

Gauge is the Diameter of the needle lumen used for venipuncture.

- If the gauge of the needle is **smaller**, the lumen of the needle would be **larger.**
- If the gauge of the needle is **larger**, the lumen of the needle would be **smaller.**

This would mean

- Higher the number (gauge), smaller the lumen (diameter)
- Lower the number (gauge), larger the lumen (diameter)

NEEDLE DESCRIPTION

Parts of a needle:

1. **A point:** A point of the needle is the part of the needle that is sharp and that functions to puncture the skin; it is the first part of the needle that comes in contact with the skin of the puncture site.

2. **Bevel:** A bevel is the opening of the needle through which the blood passes through. While performing venipuncture, the bevel of the needle should face up before inserting the needle for drawing blood.
3. **Lumen:** A lumen is the inside space of the tubular structure needle.
4. **Shaft:** Shaft is the tubular portion of the needle. Needle length (shaft) can range from 1 inch to 1 1/2 inches.
5. **Hub:** Hub is the end part of the needle. It is usually made up of plastic.

Structure of Multi-sample Needle

*   The needle has two ends.
*   The front end enters the vein.
*   Back end enters the collection tube.
*   Back end is protected with a retractable rubber sheath. The retractable rubber sheath performs the function of preventing the leaking of blood from the rear end of the needle after the front end of the needle has entered the patient's vein.

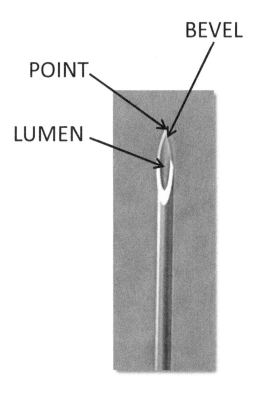

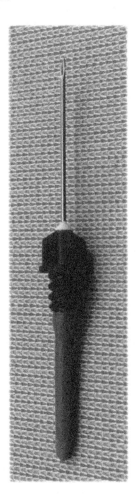

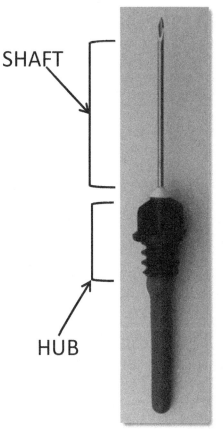

Figure 4.5 Parts of Needle

NEEDLE GAUGE

A phlebotomy technician must be familiar with what the needle gauge is and its importance in performing phlebotomy procedures. The gauge of the needle indicates the diameter (bore size) of the needle.

What is the Diameter: The diameter is a straight line that starts from one end of the circle to another end of the circle through the center.

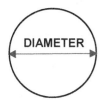

The selection of the proper gauge needle depends on factors such as the vein size, amount of blood to be collected and age of the patient. Children may have small veins as compared to adults.

- If the gauge of the needle is **smaller**, the lumen of the needle would be **larger**.
  - If a small gauge needle **that has a larger lumen** is used to perform the procedure on a smaller diameter vein, the blood sample collected may become **clotted**.
- If the gauge of the needle is **larger**, the lumen of the needle would be **smaller**.
  - If a large gauge needle **that has a smaller lumen** is used to perform the procedure on a larger diameter vein, the blood sample collected may become **hemolyzed**.

The phlebotomy technician must use the appropriate gauge needle after the patient's vein is assessed.

ANGLE AT WHICH THE NEEDLE IS INSERTED FOR BLOOD DRAWS:

a) 15 degree for a superficial vein.
b) 30 degree for a deeper vein.

GAUGE OF NEEDLE:

a) Smaller the gauge, larger the needle lumen.
b) Larger the gauge, smaller the needle lumen.

GAUGE SIZE:

a) 18 Gauge (Largest Needle Size)
b) 20 Gauge, 21 Gauge
c) 22 Gauge (Small Needle Size)
d) 23 Gauge & 25 Gauge (Winged infusion needle is also known as a butterfly needle)

Syringe

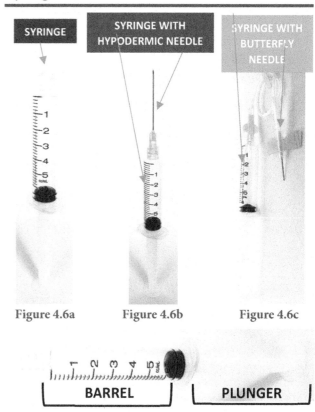

Figure 4.6a   Figure 4.6b   Figure 4.6c

Figure 4.7: Syringe

The syringe has two parts: The plunger and the barrel. The **plunger** when pulled back functions to fill the syringe and when pushed into the barrel functions to empty the syringe. The **barrel** functions to hold the content that is being collected. The front end of the syringe allows for the attachment of a needle. The needle that can be attached to the front end of the syringe depends on the procedure that is to be performed; it can be a hypodermic needle, butterfly needle, e.t.c. Syringe and needle are used in collecting blood (venipuncture) when the veins of the patient cannot withstand the suction pressure (vein collapse) of the blood collection tube. In this case, a syringe is used since the suction pressure can be controlled by the plunger of the syringe. While pulling the plunger when drawing blood, the speed of pulling the plunger should be slow. If the plunger is pulled too quickly, it may cause the vein to collapse and or the sample may become hemolyzed. After the blood is collected in the barrel of the syringe, using a transfer device the blood collected is transferred into the blood collection tube.

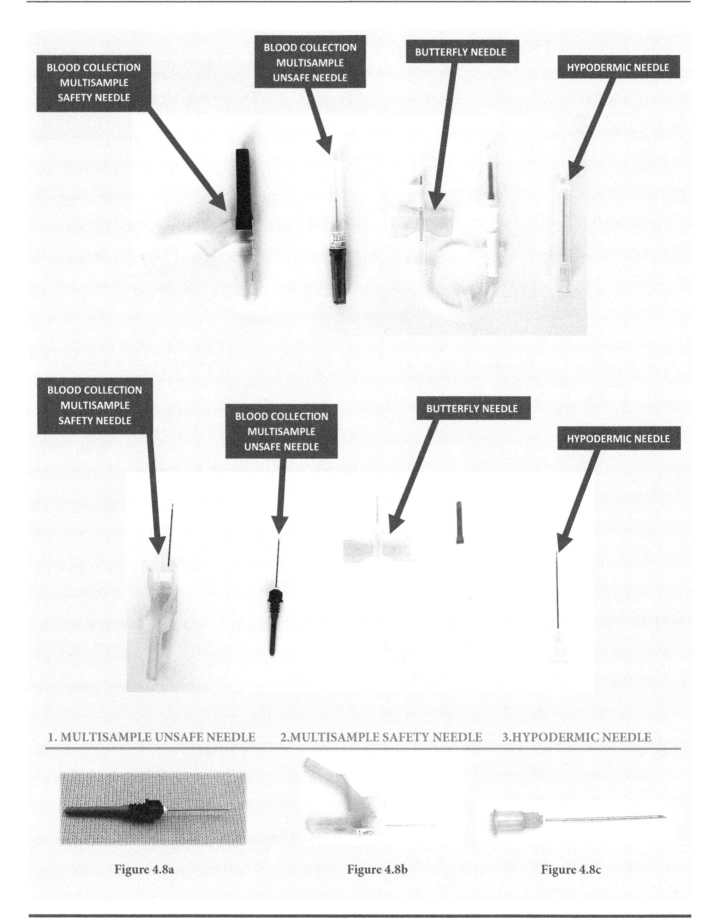

BLOOD COLLECTION MULTISAMPLE SAFETY NEEDLE

BLOOD COLLECTION MULTISAMPLE UNSAFE NEEDLE

BUTTERFLY NEEDLE

HYPODERMIC NEEDLE

BLOOD COLLECTION MULTISAMPLE SAFETY NEEDLE

BLOOD COLLECTION MULTISAMPLE UNSAFE NEEDLE

BUTTERFLY NEEDLE

HYPODERMIC NEEDLE

1. MULTISAMPLE UNSAFE NEEDLE   2.MULTISAMPLE SAFETY NEEDLE   3.HYPODERMIC NEEDLE

Figure 4.8a   Figure 4.8b   Figure 4.8c

4. BUTTERFLY OR WINGED NEEDLE

Butterfly needle is a specialized needle that has butterfly flaps (two) on either side with the needle placed in the center. It also has a tubing attached to the rear end of the needle. The flaps of the butterfly needle are used to hold the butterfly needle in place. Performing venipuncture procedure using butterfly needle allows precise placement of the needle; this occurs due to the grasp of the flaps being close to the needle. When the butterfly needle enters the vein, the blood from the vein enters the lumen of the butterfly needle and a flash of blood is seen in the tubing indicating that the needle has entered the vein. They are mostly used on patients that have small veins. The rear end of the tubing from the butterfly needle set can be attached to either an evacuated tube holder or to a syringe. Most commonly used butterfly needle gauges are 21 and 23 gauge.

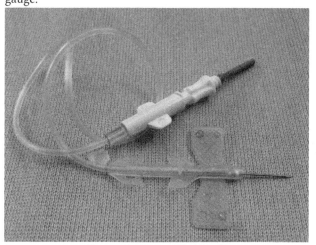

Figure 4.9 Butterfly Needle

Remember:

- If a small gauge needle **that has a larger lumen** is used to perform the procedure on a smaller diameter vein, the blood sample collected may become **clotted**.
- If a large gauge needle **that has a smaller lumen** is used to perform the procedure on a larger diameter vein, the blood sample collected may become **hemolyzed**.

The phlebotomy technician must use the appropriate gauge needle after the patient's vein is assessed.

NEEDLE HOLDER

Needle holder is the plastic holder onto which the:
- Double ended needle is screwed at one end and
- Evacuated collection tube is inserted on the other end.

- The needle holder functions to hold:
  - The needle (before and during the procedure) and
  - The collection tube in place (during the procedure).

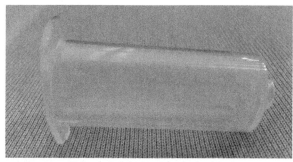

Figure 4.10 NEEDLE HOLDER

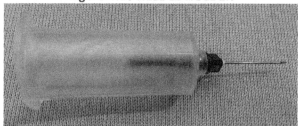

Figure 4.11 NEEDLE HOLDER WITH MULTISAMPLE NEEDLE

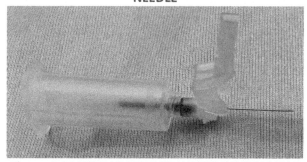

Figure 4.12 NEEDLE HOLDER WITH MULTISAMPLE SAFETY LOCK NEEDLE

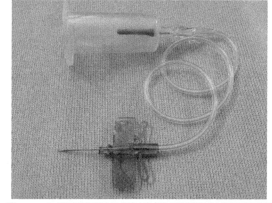

Figure 4.13 NEEDLE HOLDER WITH BUTTERFLY NEEDLE

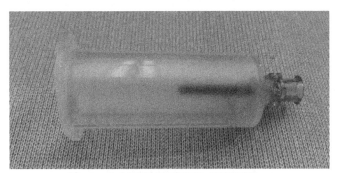

Figure 4.14 TRANSFER DEVICE

SHARPS CONTAINER

The sharps container is a red color container with a biohazard label and is available in various shapes and sizes to fit the needs of the facility. The sharps container functions to hold the sharp objects such as needles and lancets after they are used. The technique of properly disposing of the used needle is to drop the needle into the sharps container without touching the sharps container. The sharps container disposal regulations differ in each state. Follow your state regulations when disposing of the sharps container(s). The sharps container must have features such as it should be leak proof, puncture resistant, and closable. Various type of sharps are available in the market, some that are small and can be placed on the table (table top), while on the other hand there are large sharps container that are placed on the floor or are mounted on the wall. If mounted on the wall, it should be placed at such height that it is easily accessible for disposing of sharps. The sharps containers must only be filled to its recommended capacity.

Note: sharps such as needle must not be disposed into the regular waste containers or recycling containers. It must be discarded in a sharps container. For phlebotomy technicians, the objects that must be disposed of in the sharps containers are safety needles, multisample needles, hypodermic needles, lancets, syringes, butterfly needles, capillary tubes, or any other sharps. Sharps can be explained as objects that can cut or scrape the skin or other body parts. Remember, the purpose of using sharps container is to protect people from getting injured from the sharps. Hence, phlebotomy technician must not try to bend or break the needle since this can injure them. Also, make sure that once the used needle is disposed into the sharps container, no attempts should be made to withdraw the needle from the sharps container.

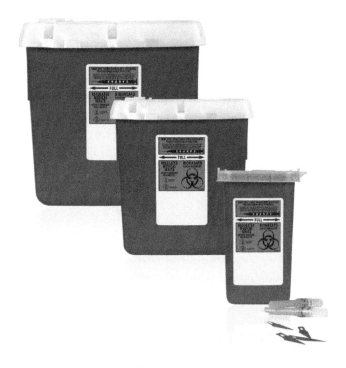

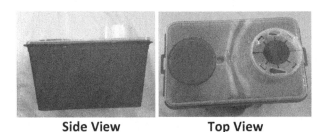

Side View   **Top View**

Figure 4.15

EVACUATED BLOOD COLLECTION TUBES

The blood collection tubes used for collection of blood during venipuncture procedures are known as evacuated blood collection tubes. The evacuated tubes are pre-filled with vacuum and are sealed with a top rubber stopper. The presence of vacuum in the tube creates a negative pressure within the blood collection tube. When the front end of the needle is in the vein, and the rear end of the needle is inserted into the tube, the tube creates a suction-like effect (due to the presence of pre-filled vacuum) onto the vein assisting the blood from the vein to be collected into the tube.

The tube:

1. **Physical Form:** The evacuated blood collection tubes are made up of glass or plastic.
2. **Sizes:** They are available in different sizes and are selected as per their requirement.
3. **Types:** They are color coded and can be distinguished by the color of the rubber stopper sealing the tube.
4. **Contents:** Additives may be present or absent.

When using the evacuated blood collection tubes, the tubes must be properly selected as per the requisition form. The tube must be checked for any manufacturing defects, damages or expiration. The rubber stopper must also be carefully checked for any defects, since a defective rubber stopper may cause the prefilled vacuum to escape from the tube.

TUBE INVERSION TECHNIQUE

Tubes must be gently inverted as per recommended guidelines when collecting blood in a tube that contains the additive. The reason for inverting the tube several times is to appropriately mix the blood and the additive. The inversions must be performed as per the recommended number of inversions for the color coded tube for e.g. 5 – 8 times. When performing the inversion technique ensure that the inversions are not forceful, since doing so may cause the blood sample to undergo hemolysis. On the other hand, if the inversions are not properly performed, the blood sample may clot.

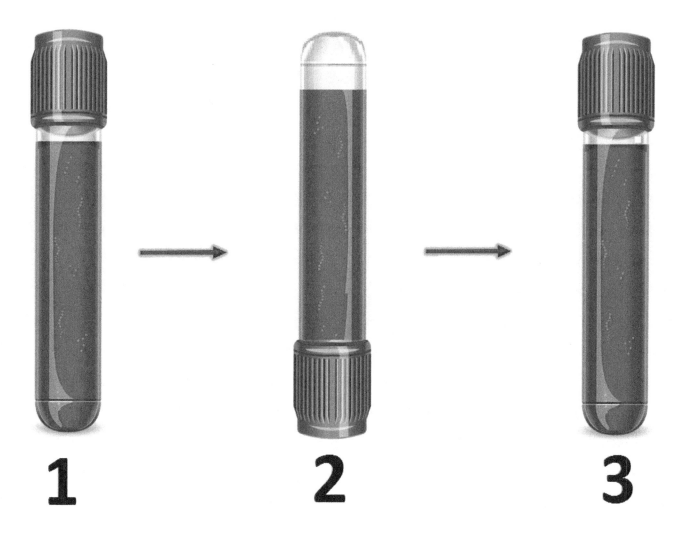

1 COMPLETE INVERSION

Figure 4.16

94

BLOOD SPECIMENS IN PHLEBOTOMY

The type of test that will be performed on the specimen collected determines the type of specimen that is to be collected by performing the phlebotomy procedure. When collecting blood, the phlebotomy technician collects the blood into the blood collection tube. The blood collected is the **whole blood specimen**. If a **plasma specimen** or **serum specimen** is required, the following steps must be performed.

For plasma specimen:

1. Collect the whole blood into the specified color collection tube.
2. Next, centrifuge the collection tube for 15 minutes.
3. After the centrifuging process is over, remove the tube from the centrifuge machine. The tube will have a top yellow layer of fluid. This yellow layer is the plasma. Using a pipette transfer the plasma from the tube to a vial.

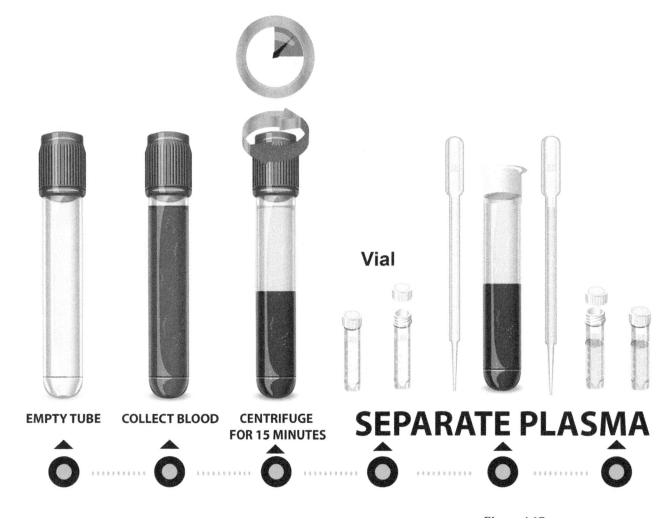

Vial

EMPTY TUBE **COLLECT BLOOD** **CENTRIFUGE FOR 15 MINUTES** **SEPARATE PLASMA**

Figure 4.17a

For serum specimen:

1. Collect the whole blood into the specified color collection tube.
2. Let the collection tube sit for 30-45 minutes.
3. Next, centrifuge the collection tube for 15 minutes.
4. After the centrifuging process is over, remove the tube from the centrifuge machine. The tube will have a top yellow layer of fluid. This yellow layer is the serum. Using a pipette transfer the serum from the tube to a vial.

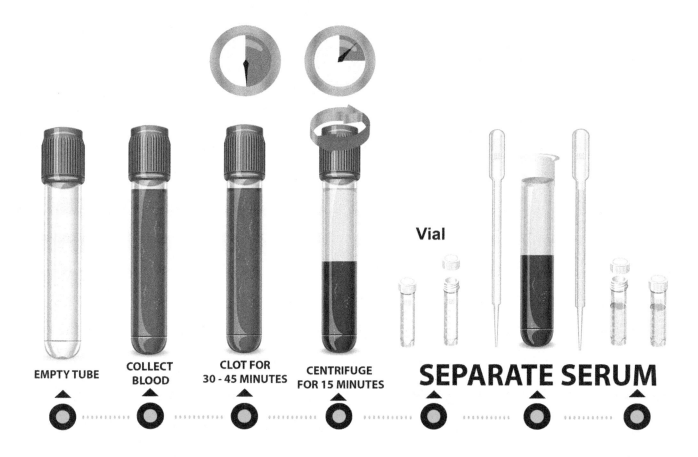

EMPTY TUBE   **COLLECT BLOOD**   **CLOT FOR 30 - 45 MINUTES**   **CENTRIFUGE FOR 15 MINUTES**   **SEPARATE SERUM**

Figure 4.17b

TUBE ADDITIVES

Tube additive are a small proportion of an additive that is added to the tube by the manufacturer. **The addition of the additive to the tube serves the function of either;**

1. Inhibiting (**stopping**) the process of coagulation of blood after collection or
2. Initiating (**starting or activating**) the process of coagulation or
3. Separating the blood layers after spinning the tube in the centrifuge.

Coagulation is a process that causes the blood to change its form from liquid to a semisolid or gel-like substance also known as a clot. Coagulation is sometimes also known as clotting.

TYPES OF ADDITIVES

- **Anticoagulant:** Inhibiting coagulation.
- **Clot activator:** Initiating coagulation.
- **Thixotropic gel:** Separating the blood layers after spinning the tube in the centrifuge.

ANTICOAGULANTS

Anticoagulants inhibit the blood clotting (coagulation) process, thereby letting the blood collected in the blood collection tube stay in the liquid form.

Types of anticoagulants

- EDTA (Ethylene-diamine-tetra-acetic-acid)
- Sodium Citrate
- Potassium Oxalate
- SPS (Sodium Polyanethole Sulfonate)
- Heparin
- Sodium Fluoride
- Lithium Idoacetate

CLOT ACTIVATORS

Clot activator is a type of additive that is added to the tube to activate the clotting mechanism. They enhance the process of clotting or coagulation. For e.g **Silica**

THIXOTROPIC GEL

The thixotropic gel is an additive that is added to the tube to separate the layers of blood. The blood collected in such tubes are spun in the centrifuge which leads to the gel separating the layers of the blood.

BLOOD COLLECTION COLOR CODED TUBES

Tube:	•Plastic Red & Glass Red
Tube:	•Yellow (Sterile)
Tube:	•Yellow (Non-Sterile)
Tube:	•Light Blue
Tube:	•Gray
Tube:	•Gold
Tube:	•Lavender
Tube:	•Light green
Tube:	•Green
Tube:	•Royal blue
Tube:	•Orange
Tube:	•Tan
Tube:	•Pink

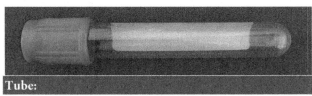

Tube:
Plastic Red & Glass Red (Blood clotting time 30 minutes)
Additive:
Plastic: Clot activators - Glass: No additive
Specimen:
Serum
Laboratory Uses:
Chemistry, Serology, Immunology, & Blood Bank

Tube:
Yellow (Sterile)
Additive:
SPS (Sodium Polyanethole Sulfonate)
Specimen:
Whole blood
Laboratory Uses:
Blood and bodily fluid cultures

Tube:
Yellow (Non-Sterile)
Additive:
Acid Citrate Dextrose (ACD)
Specimen:
Whole blood
Laboratory Uses:

DNA, human leukocyte antigen phenotyping (HLA), and paternity testing.

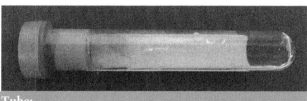

Tube:
Light Blue
Additive:
Sodium Citrate
Specimen:
Plasma
Laboratory Uses:
Coagulation studies:
PT, PTT, and fibrinogen

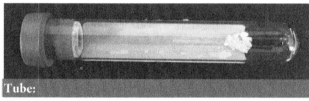

Tube:
Gray
Additive:
Potassium Oxalate/Sodium Fluoride
Specimen:
Plasma
Laboratory Uses:
Glucose levels, Blood alcohol level, GTT, Lactate, and Bicarbonate

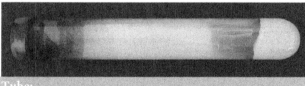

Tube:
Gold Stopper. Also called SSTs (Serum Separation Tubes)
Additive:
Clot activator and gel
Specimen:
Serum
Laboratory Uses:
Chemistry (glucose, BUN)

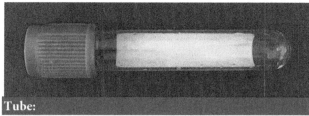

Tube:
Lavender
Additive:
EDTA K_2, EDTA K_3
Specimen:
Whole blood
Laboratory Uses:
Hematology studies: CBC, WBC count, Hemoglobin, Hematocrit, Platelet count, Erythrocyte Sedimentation Rate (ESR), *RBC, Reticulocyte, and differential count*.

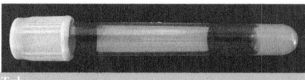

Tube:
Light green or green/gray stopper. Also called as a PST or plasma separation tube.
Additive:
Lithium Heparin and gel
Specimen:
Plasma
Laboratory Uses:
Plasma determinations in chemistry studies

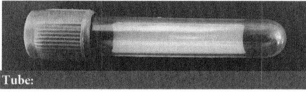

Tube:
Green
Additive:
Sodium Heparin or Lithium Heparin
Specimen:
Specimen: Plasma
Laboratory Uses:
Chemistry Testing-Stat chemistry tests, glucose, ammonia, and electrolytes

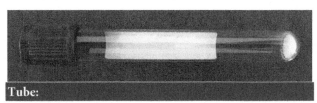

Tube:

Royal blue

Additive:

Sodium Heparin **or** Sodium EDTA **or** No Additive

Specimen:

Plasma or serum

Laboratory Uses:

Chemistry trace elements: Toxicology trace metals, lead, and nutrition analysis

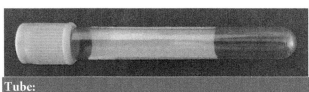

Tube:

Pink

Additive:

K_2 EDTA (Potassium EDTA)

Specimen:

Whole blood or plasma

Laboratory Uses:

Hematology, Blood bank compatibility testing, and antibody screening.

Tube:

Orange Stopper

Additive:

Thrombin (clot activator) or Thrombin (clot activator) with gel

Specimen:

Serum

Laboratory Uses:

STAT serum chemistries

Tube:

Tan

Additive:

K_2EDTA (Potassium EDTA)

Specimen:

Plasma

Laboratory Uses:

Lead

ORDER OF DRAW

The phlebotomy technician collects blood in a specified evacuated blood collection tube by following the orders in the requisition form. When a multi-sample draw is requested, the phlebotomy technician will be required to fill multiple blood collection tubes to fulfill the requisition ordered. When collecting blood in multiple blood collection tubes, the correct order of draw must be performed. This would mean that the standard order must be followed to fill the blood collection tube. The correct order of draw is done to prevent contamination of the tubes by mixing of additive(s) from one tube to another. This may not only cause inaccurate results but may also result in misdiagnosis. Therefore, it is important that the correct order of draw is followed when obtaining blood into multiple tubes.

Correct order of draw:

1. **Blood culture tube** (sterile) or Yellow SPS
2. **Coagulation tube** (light blue top; sodium citrate)
3. **Serum** tube without clot activator (glass red top) and with clot activator (plastic red top), Serum Separator Tubes (SSTs)
4. **Plasma Separator Tubes** (PSTs) with Heparin tube and Heparin Tube (green top).
5. **EDTA** tube without gel separator (lavender top, Pink top) and EDTA tube with Plasma Preparation Tubes (PPTs) (white top)
6. **Glycolytic inhibitor** (gray top)

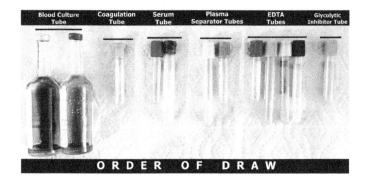

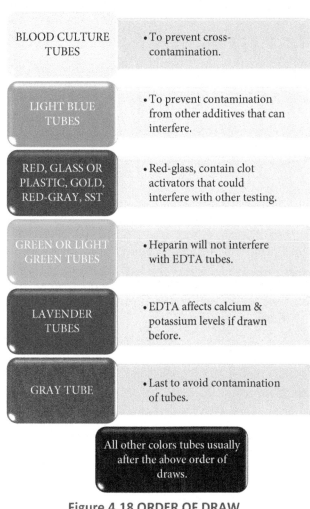

Figure 4.18 ORDER OF DRAW
Your Brother Robert Gave Lovely Gifts
Yellow: Light Blue : Red : Green : Lavender : Gray

DERMAL PUNCTURE

Dermal puncture is a procedure that involves making an incision on the skin to obtain blood. **Dermal puncture** is also known as **Skin Puncture** and **Capillary Puncture**. The device used to create the incision on the skin is called the "**Lancet**". The lancet comes in various forms such as trigger button lancet, pen lancet, twist top lancet, etc. Most commonly used lancets are the trigger button lancet. The procedure of using the trigger button lancet is to place the tip of the lancet onto the surface of the skin, followed by pushing the trigger button on the superior surface of the lancet, this pushing action activates the sharp within the lancet to spring to the surface of the skin causing a cut to the surface of the skin that leads to bleeding. The blood obtained by this method is the capillary blood.

The dermal puncture is a procedure chosen:
- when the blood sample required are to be collected from the capillary, or
- when other methods of blood draws are not recommended, or
- when the amount of blood required is minimal in quantity.

Dermal puncture is most commonly performed
- to check the blood glucose levels.
- on infants for neonatal screening.
- on patients with vascular conditions that contraindicate venipuncture.
- on patients with fragile veins.

Dermal puncture procedure should not be performed if the following test is to be performed
- Blood Cultures
- Erythrocytes Sedimentation Rates
- Coagulation Tests
- any test that requires large volume of samples

UNDERSTANDING CAPILLARY BLOOD

Capillary blood is a mixture of:
- Arterial Blood
- Venous Blood

The capillary blood consists of the blood from the arterial system, which would be the oxygenated blood and other nutrients, while on the other hand, it would also consist of the blood from the venous system, and that would be the deoxygenated blood and other waste substances or materials. The capillary is the connection between the arterial system and the venous system. Its main function is to provide oxygen and nutrients to the tissue and collected carbon dioxide and waste substances from the tissue.

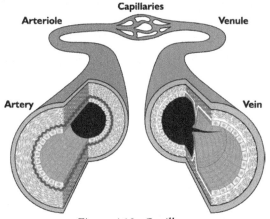

Figure 4.19a Capillary

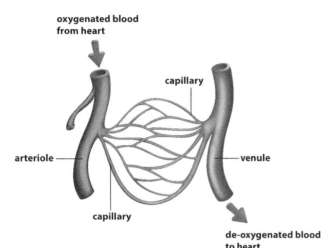

oxygenated blood
from heart

capillary

arteriole

venule

capillary

de-oxygenated blood
to heart

Figure 4.19b Capillary

EQUIPMENT AND SUPPLIES REQUIRED FOR DERMAL PUNCTURE

Glucose Testing

- Lancet
- Alcohol Pad
- Cotton
- Gauze or Bandage
- Sharps container
- Gloves
- Glucose Test Strip
- Glucose Analyzer Machine

Capillary Tube Blood Collection

- Lancet
- Capillary Tube
- Alcohol Pad
- Cotton
- Gauze or Bandage
- Sharps container
- Gloves
- Hematocrit centrifuge
- Clay sealant

Bleeding Time Test

- Lancet
- Alcohol Pad
- Cotton
- Gauze or Bandage
- Sharps container
- Gloves
- Blood Pressure Set
- Timer

- Filter Paper

Neonatal Screening

- Gloves
- Lancet
- Alcohol Pads
- Gauze Pads
- Sharps Container
- Bandages
- Newborn Screening Cards
- Storage bag
- Other equipment and supplies may be required.

CONTAINERS

When performing dermal puncture, the volume of blood

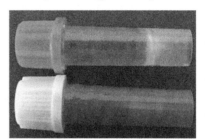

collected is lower than that of the volume of blood collected on a venipuncture. To collect such less volume of blood, **capillary blood collection small plastic tubes** are used. These small plastic containers or tubes are used to collect the blood sample from a heel or finger puncture. It has two parts: a cap and a container. Unscrewing the cap is required to fill the blood sample into the container by directly dropping the blood into the container. Once the blood has been collected into the **capillary blood collection small plastic tube**, it must be sealed by recapping the container.

CAPILLARY TUBES

Obtaining blood samples directly into the **capillary blood collection small plastic tubes** is not always required. Some procedures may require the blood to be collected in a capillary tube. A capillary tube is a **thin cylindrical glass tube with two ends.** Both the ends of the capillary tube are open. Blood is collected from one end, while the other end is sealed once the tube is filled with the required amount of capillary blood obtained by a dermal puncture.

There are two types of capillary tubes available:

1. **Heparinized Capillary Tubes:** Heparinized tube has a **red color band** across its circumference that can be seen towards the bottom portion of the tube.

2. **Non-Heparinized Capillary Tubes:** Non-Heparinized tube has a **blue color band** across its

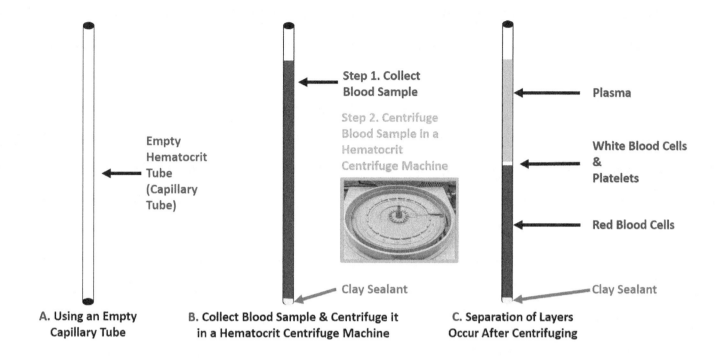

A. Using an Empty
Capillary Tube

B. Collect Blood Sample & Centrifuge it
in a Hematocrit Centrifuge Machine

C. Separation of Layers
Occur After Centrifuging

Figure 4.20 Capillary Sample Processing

circumference that can be seen towards the bottom portion of the tube.

To fill the tube, the front end of the capillary tube is to be placed in close proximity to the drop of blood (on the skin after dermal puncture). When the front open end of the tube touches the drop of blood, the drop of blood is suctioned into the capillary tube due to the capillary action of the tube, once the blood is collected into the tube, the other end of the tube must be blocked manually with the phlebotomy technicians fingertip (gloved hand). Continue the step of collecting the blood by touching the drop of blood to the front open end of the tube until a required amount of sample is collected. Finally, the capillary tube must be sealed with a clay sealant.

When to block and unblock the rear end of the capillary tube:

To fill blood into the capillary tube

- **Unblock**, the rear end of the capillary tube, to
  - Allow the blood to flow into the capillary tube or
  - If an air bubble enters the capillary tube, unblock the rear end of the tube and tilt the front end of the capillary tube in a slightly downward direction to remove the air bubble from the front end of the capillary tube.

To stop the blood from flowing out of the rear end of the capillary tube

- **Block** the rear end of the tube by placing the finger of the gloved hand. The blocking maneuver creates a barrier and does not allow the blood within the capillary tube to flow within the tube. Hence, the blocking maneuver can be utilized to control the flow of blood within the capillary tube.

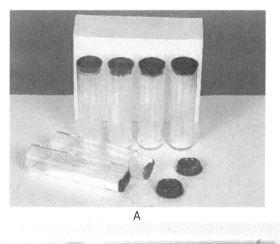

A

B

Figure 4.21 Capillary Tubes

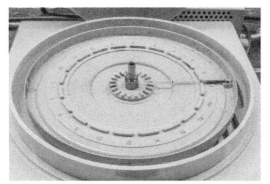
Figure 4.22a Hematocrit Centrifuge Machine

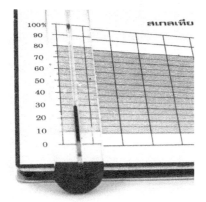
Figure 4.22b Microhematocrit Tube Reader

LANCET

Dermal puncture is a procedure that involves making an incision on the skin to obtain blood. The device used to create the incision onto the skin is called the "**Lancet**". The lancet comes in various forms such as trigger button lancet, pen lancet, twist top lancet, etc. Most commonly used lancets are the trigger button lancet. The procedure of using the trigger button lancet is to place the tip of the lancet onto the surface of the skin, followed by pushing the trigger button on the superior surface of the lancet, this pushing action activates the sharp within the lancet to spring to the surface of the skin causing a cut to the surface of the skin that leads to bleeding. The lancet must be disposed into the sharps container after its use. The lancets are also available in a variety of gauges. The gauge select depends on the depth of incision that is required. *Note: never perform an incision over a bone.*

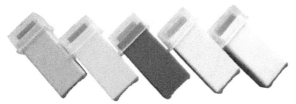
Figure 4.23 Lancet

WARMING DEVICE

When performing heel puncture on infants, a warming device is required to warm the area. This is done to increase the flow of blood in the area. Prior to performing the dermal puncture, the warming device is placed in contact with the heel for 3 to 5 minutes in duration. The temperature should not exceed the recommended temperature. Checking the facility procedure manual is crucial prior to performing such procedures. If a warming device is not to be used, another device or method may be recommended by the facility to warm the heel; this may be found in the facility procedure manual or other resources.

INCISION WIDTH AND DEPTH

Width
- Should not exceed 2.4 mm

Depth
- Should not exceed 2.0 mm in infant heels

DERMAL PUNCTURE SITES

Puncture should be done on the palmar surface of the distal segments.
- Middle finger (non-dominant hand)
- Ring finger (non-dominant hand)

Puncture should be:
- Perpendicular to the fingerprints.

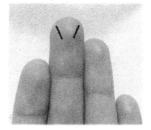 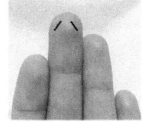

Correct   Incorrect
Figure 4.24
The incision should be made perpendicular to the finger whorls.

DERMAL PUNCTURE SITE SELECTION

Newborn to 12 months:
- Medial or lateral side of the heel.

More than 12 months to adult:
- Middle or ring finger, care should be taken to avoid an incision on the bone.

DERMAL PUNCTURE ORDER OF DRAW

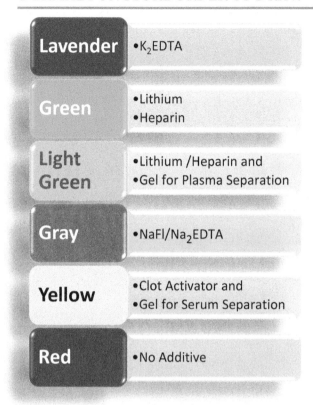

Lavender	•K_2EDTA
Green	•Lithium •Heparin
Light Green	•Lithium /Heparin and •Gel for Plasma Separation
Gray	•NaFl/Na_2EDTA
Yellow	•Clot Activator and •Gel for Serum Separation
Red	•No Additive

Figure 4.25
Larry Gave Lovely **Girl** Yellow **Rose**
Lavender : Green : Light Green : **Gray** : Yellow : **Red**

CENTRIFUGE

To obtain a plasma or serum sample, the blood in the tube must be spun in a centrifuge machine. A centrifuge machine is a device that spins and uses the centrifugal force to separate the heavier and lighter particles from each other. The centrifugal force causes the lighter particles to move towards the top and the heavier particles to move to the bottom.

Components of a centrifuge machine are:

Rotor

The rotor is the part of the centrifuge machine that rotates at a set speed. The rotations are referred to as the rotations per minute. The rotations per minute can be set as per the requirement.

Motor

The motor is the part of the centrifuge machine that causes the centrifuge unit to function.

Imbalance detector

Imbalance detector is the part of the centrifuge machine that detects the imbalance of mass placed in the centrifuge machine. If the load is not balanced properly, the machine may not operate.

Tachometer

The tachometer is the part of the centrifuge machine that displays the speed at which rotor rotates.

Safety lid

Safety lid is the part of the centrifuge machine that covers the centrifuge machine.

Braking system

The braking system is the part of the centrifuge machine that decelerates the machine from spinning.

Note: before you operate a centrifuge unit, make sure to read the operating manual of the unit. The operation manual will provide details on the operating procedures of the machine.

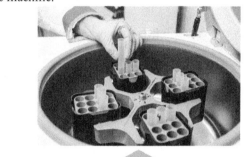

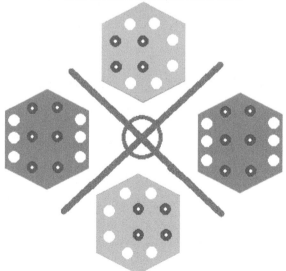

◉ = Tubes

Figure 4.26a Balancing Centrifuge Machine
Tube loads (specimens) are balanced on the opposite side

PROCEDURE

1. Check to verify the type of sample that will be centrifuged.
2. Identify the speed and duration at which the sample is to be centrifuged.

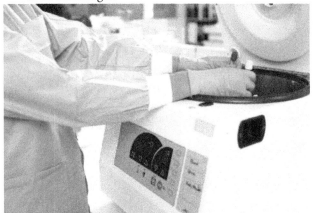

Figure 4.26b Centrifuge Machine

3. Place the samples into the rotor. If the samples do not have the same mass, place samples with the same mass on opposite sides of the rotor. If the machine is not properly balanced, the machine will start making noises and set the unit to vibrate.

4. Once the samples are placed/loaded, secure the rotor lid properly, close the centrifuge lid and set the required speed and time at which the sample is to be spun.
5. When ready, press the "Start" button and wait for the unit to reach the required speed.
6. When the spinning cycle is over, and the rotor has completely stopped spinning, unlock the centrifuge lid and carefully remove the samples.

Specimen Processing

When blood specimens are obtained, they may either be required to:

1. **Clot** and then **Centrifuge** or
2. **Directly Centrifuge** after collection.

Depending on what is required. The specimen after being centrifuged must be aliquoted. Aliquoting means removing the serum or plasma from the centrifuged specimen using a transfer pipette into an appropriate recommended cryovial.

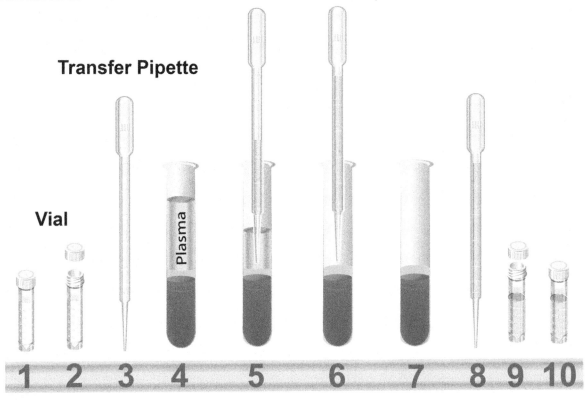

Figure 4.27 Aliquoting

CHAPTER 4
END OF CHAPTER REVIEW QUESTIONS
Question Set 1: Match the following

Column A	Column B
____Types of Blood Specimen Collected	A. Anticoagulant, Clot Activator, Thixotropic Gel
____Gray	B. EDTA K$_2$
____Light Green	C. Sodium Citrate
____Light Blue	D. Types of Anticoagulants
____Medial or Lateral Side Of Heel	E. Lithium Heparin and Gel
____Rotor	F. Whole Blood, Serum, and Plasma
____Types of Additives	G. Dermal Puncture Site Selection; New Born To 12 Months
____Lavender Tube	H. Dermal Puncture
____EDTA (Ethylene-Diamine-Tetra-Acetic-Acid, Sodium Citrate, Heparin, and Sodium Fluoride)	I. Centrifuge Machine Part
____Patients Prone to Develop Venous Thrombosis	J. Potassium Oxalate and Sodium Fluoride

Question Set 2: Essay Questions
1. List the equipment used in glucose testing.
2. Explain in brief about latex sensitivity.
3. Explain uses and parts of a multisample needle.
4. Explain in brief about sharps container.
5. Explain the procedure of tube inversion.
6. What are the uses of additives in blood collection tubes?
7. List the names of anticoagulants.

Question Set 3: Fill in the blanks
1. Fill in the names of the equipment and supplies required for Evacuated Tube Method (phlebotomy)?
   a. Needle (Safe or Unsafe Needle)
   b. _____
   c. _____
   d. Alcohol Pad
   e. Cotton
   f. Gauze
   g. Bandage
   h. Sharps container
   i. Gloves
   j. _____
2. In a dermal puncture procedure, the width should not exceed _____ mm.
3. In a dermal puncture procedure the depth should not exceed _____mm.
4. The content of the most commonly used alcohol pads are 70% _____ alcohol, an antiseptic, to cleanse the skin before a venipuncture.
5. Tube: Plastic Red & Glass Red (Blood clotting time 30 minutes)
   Additive: Plastic: Clot activators Glass: No additive
   Specimen: Serum
   Laboratory Uses: _____
   _____
6. Tube: Yellow (Sterile)
   Additive: _____
   SSTs (Serum Separation Tubes)
   Specimen: Whole blood
   Laboratory Uses: Blood and bodily fluid cultures

7. Tube: Yellow (Non-Sterile)
   Additive: Acid citrate dextrose additives (ACD)
   Specimen: _____
   _____
   Laboratory Uses: HLA phenotyping, DNA, and paternity testing.
8. Tube: Light Blue
   Additive: _____
   _____
   Specimen: Plasma
   Laboratory Uses: _____
   _____
   _____
9. Tube: _____
   _____
   Additive: Potassium Oxalate and Sodium Fluoride
   Specimen: Plasma
   Laboratory Uses: Glucose levels, Blood alcohol level, GTT, Lactate, and Bicarbonate
10. Tube: _____
    _____
    Additive: Clot activator/polymer gel
    Specimen: Serum
    Laboratory Uses: Chemistry (glucose and BUN)
11. Tube: Lavender
    Additive: _____
    _____
    Specimen: _____
    _____
    Laboratory Uses: Hematology studies: CBC, WBC count, Hemoglobin,
    Hematocrit, Platelet count, Reticulocyte count, and differential count
12. Tube: Light green. Also called as a PST or plasma separation tube.
    Additive: _____
    _____
    Specimen: Plasma
    Laboratory Uses: _____
    _____
13. Tube: Green

Additive: Heparin (Sodium/Lithium)
Specimen: _____
_____
Laboratory Uses: _____
_____
14. Tube: _____
    _____
    Additive: Sodium Heparin or Sodium EDTA
    Specimen: Plasma or serum
    Laboratory Uses: Chemistry trace elements: Toxicology trace metals, lead, and nutrition analysis
15. Tube: Orange Stopper
    Additive: Thrombin (clot activator)
    Specimen: _____
    _____
    Laboratory Uses: _____
    _____
16. Tube: Tan
    Additive: Potassium EDTA
    Specimen: _____
    _____
    Laboratory Uses: _____
    _____
17. Tube: Pink
    Additive: _____
    _____
    Specimen: Whole blood or plasma
    Laboratory Uses: _____
    _____

(1) Which of the following is not a part of the Evacuated Tube Method (phlebotomy)?
(a) Needle (Safe or Unsafe Needle)
(b) Tube Holder
(c) Tube
(d) Alcohol Pad
(e) Cotton
(f) Capillary Tube
(g) Gauze
(h) Bandage
(i) Sharps Container
(j) Gloves
(k) Tourniquet

(2) Which of the following is not a part of the Winged Infusion Method (phlebotomy)?
(a) Butter Fly Needle
(b) Tube Holder
(c) Tube
(d) Alcohol Pad
(e) Cotton
(f) Gauze
(g) Test Strip
(h) Bandage
(i) Sharps Container
(j) Gloves
(k) Tourniquet

(3) Which of the following is not a part of the Syringe Method (phlebotomy)?
(a) Needle & Syringe
(b) Transfer Device
(c) Tube Holder
(d) Tube
(e) Alcohol Pad
(f) Cotton
(g) Gauze
(h) Bandage
(i) Sharps Container
(j) Gloves
(k) Tourniquet

(4) Which of the following is not a part of the Glucose Testing (phlebotomy)?
(a) Lancet
(b) Alcohol Pad
(c) Glucose Analyzer Machine
(d) Tube Holder
(e) Gauze or Bandage
(f) Sharps Container
(g) Gloves
(h) Glucose Test Strip

(5) Which of the following is not a part of the Capillary Test (phlebotomy)?
(a) Capillary Tube
(b) Alcohol Pad
(c) Cotton
(d) Gauze or Bandage
(e) Sharps Container
(f) Gloves
(g) Centrifuge

(6) Which of the following is not a part of the Bleeding Time Test (phlebotomy)?
(a) Lancet
(b) Alcohol Pad
(c) Cotton
(d) Test Strip
(e) Gauze or Bandage
(f) Sharps Container
(g) Gloves
(h) Blood Pressure Set
(i) Timer Filter Paper

(7) Which of the following in an incorrect statement about MULTISAMPLE NEEDLES?
(a) They come in various lengths
(b) They come in various gauges
(c) Gauge is the diameter of the needle lumen
(d) Smaller the gauge, smaller the lumen

(8) Which of the following is not an anticoagulant?
(a) EDTA (Ethylene-Diamine-Tetra-Acetic Acid)
(b) Thixotropic gel
(c) Potassium Oxalate
(d) SPS (Sodium Polyanethole Sulfonate)
(e) Heparin
(f) Sodium Fluoride
(g) Lithium Idoacetate

(9) Incorrect order of draw may not cause:
   (a) Increase in coagulation time
   (b) Contaminated Blood Culture Sample
   (c) Inaccurate Test Results
   (d) Inaccurate bleeding time

(10) Coagulation studies are performed in the following tube:
   (a) Light green
   (b) Yellow
   (c) Red
   (d) Light blue

Question Set 5: Rearrange the information provided in a correct order

1. **Correct Order of Draw for Venipuncture**
_____ Coagulation tube (e.g. light blue top tubes)
_____ Glycolytic inhibitor tube (e.g. gray top tubes)
_____ Serum tube with or without clot activator, with or without gel (e.g. red, gold, or speckle-top tubes)
_____ EDTA tube with or without gel separator (e.g. lavender top tubes)
_____ Heparin tube with or without gel plasma separator (e.g. green top tubes)
_____ Blood culture tube

2. **Correct Order of Draw for Dermal puncture**
_____ Light Green
_____ Gray
_____ Yellow
_____ Red
_____ Lavender
_____ Green

Question Set 6: True or False (T/F)

1) While performing phlebotomy, the phlebotomist can place the phlebotomy tray on the patient's bed.
TRUE OR FALSE

2) The tourniquet should not be left on the patient's arm for more than 60 seconds.
TRUE OR FALSE

3) Alternative antiseptics used are iodine, chlorhexidine gluconate, or benzalkonium chloride.
TRUE OR FALSE

4) Using a smaller gauge needle on a smaller diameter vein may cause hemolysis of the sample.
TRUE OR FALSE

5) If performing phlebotomy using the syringe method, the speed of pulling back on the plunger of the syringe should be quick to draw the blood.
TRUE OR FALSE

6) The red band on the capillary tube indicates non-heparinized tube.
TRUE OR FALSE

7) A gray top tube contains heparin for testing glucose levels.
TRUE OR FALSE

8) A pink top tube contains thrombin for blood bank compatibility testing.
TRUE OR FALSE

9) A lavender top tube contains EDTA K_2 for hematology studies.
TRUE OR FALSE

CLINICAL

CHAPTER 5: PHLEBOTOMY CLINICAL SKILLS

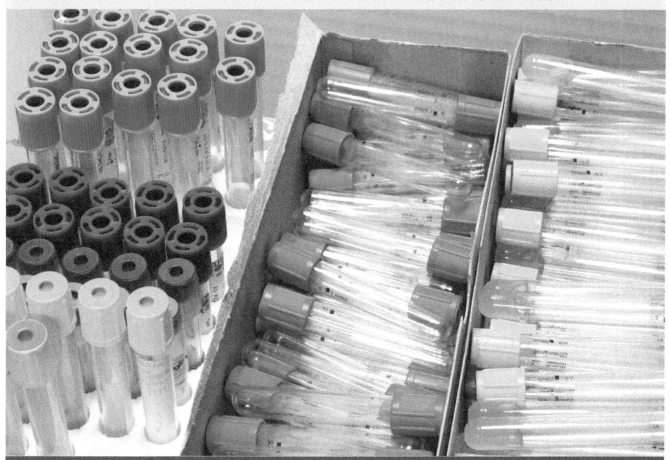

LEARNING OBJECTIVES

At the end of this chapter the student will be able to describe in brief:

Competency Checklist 5.1: Gloves Removal

Competency Checklist 5.2: Bleeding Time Test

Competency Checklist 5.3: Glucose Testing

Competency Checklist 5.4: Capillary Tube Blood Collection Procedure

Competency Checklist 5.5: Preparing Blood Smear

Competency Checklist 5.6: Venipuncture using a Multisample Needle (Method)

Competency Checklist 5.7: Venipuncture using a Winged Infusion Or Butterfly Needle (Method)

Competency Checklist 5.8: Venipuncture using a Syringe and Needle (Method)

COMPETENCY CHECKLIST 5.1: GLOVES REMOVAL

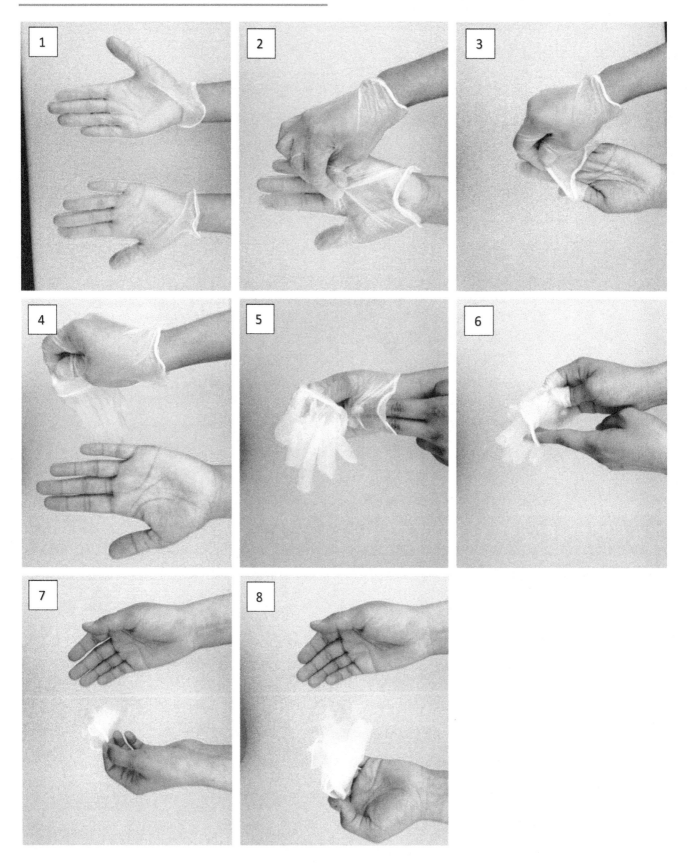

COMPETENCY CHECKLIST 5.2: BLEEDING TIME TEST

PREPARATION PHASE

1. Verifying Physician's Order.

- Depending on the facility, the phlebotomy technician might be required to read the requisition form first before proceeding to perform the procedure.
- The requisition form provides the phlebotomy technician the information about the type of procedure that is to be performed, the patient's information and other information relevant to the procedure. Therefore, read the requisition form correctly.

2. Greeting, identifying yourself, & identifying the patient (full name & date of birth).

- Greeting your patient should be done as part of work ethics. Greet and identify yourself to the patient.
- Identify patient by asking the patient's name and date of birth. More identifiers may be required according to the policy of the facility.
- Identifying the patient is a crucial step of the procedure, as improper identification may lead to potential medical errors.

3. Assembling equipment and supplies.

- Gather all the equipment and supplies required for performing the procedure.

4. Washing hands/donning PPE.

- Washing hands are performed as part of standard precautions.
- Select appropriate size gloves and don gloves.

5. Explaining procedure to the patient.

- Explaining the procedure prepares the patient for the procedure.
- The patient has the right to know about the procedure that they will be going through. Finally receive the consent from the patient for the procedure.

6. Positioning patient comfortably.

- Make sure that the patient is in a comfortable position, since some positions may compromise the procedure.

7. Checking to review if the patient is on medication or dietary restrictions.

- Check for any medication (aspirin, warfarin or heparin or others) or dietary restrictions; as some medications may increase the bleeding time.

- Follow your facility policy if the patient is on medication before the procedure is performed.
- Check if any dietary restrictions are to be followed before the procedure is performed.

PROCEDURE PHASE

SITE SELECTION

8. Selecting incision site.

- Incision site should be carefully selected.
- **Site:** Anterior surface of the forearm distal to the elbow.

Note: Follow the facility guidelines.

9. Disinfecting site with isopropyl alcohol.

- Disinfect site by appropriately cleansing the site using 70% isopropyl alcohol prep pad.
- Let the site air-dry.

10. Applying blood pressure cuff.

    o Apply blood pressure cuff onto the patient's arm and inflate the blood pressure cuff to 40 mm Hg.

11. Positioning the device onto the palmar surface of the forearm.

- Performing incision at the site.
- Wiping the first drop of blood. Start timing.

12. Blotting blood at 30-second intervals until bleeding stops.

- Blot blood with a filter paper at 30-second interval and keep recording until the bleeding completely stops.

13. Removing blood pressure cuff.

14. Applying bandage on the incision site.

15. Disposing of sharps into a sharps container.

GLOVE REMOVAL, DISPOSAL AND HAND HYGIENE

16. Removing gloves using the proper technique of glove removal.

17. Disposing of gloves and other supplies into their appropriate containers.

18. Washing hands using the proper technique of hand washing.

DOCUMENTATION

19. Documenting the procedure electronically or manually.

- Follow your facility policy on documenting the procedure.

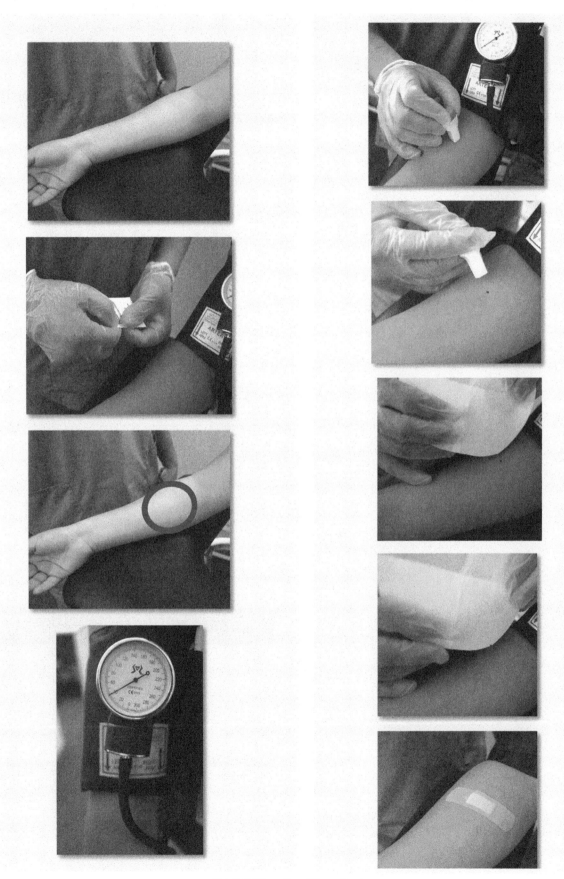

Fig 5.2 Bleeding Time Test

COMPETENCY CHECKLIST 5.3: GLUCOSE TESTING

PREPARATION PHASE

1. Verifying Physician's Order.

- Depending on the facility, the phlebotomy technician might be required to read the requisition form first before proceeding to perform the procedure.
- The requisition form provides the phlebotomy technician the information about the type of procedure that is to be performed, the patient's information and other information relevant to the procedure. Therefore, read the requisition form correctly.

2. Greeting, identifying yourself, & identifying the patient (full name & date of birth).

- Greeting your patient should be done as part of work ethics. Greet and identify yourself to the patient.
- Identify patient by asking the patient's name and date of birth. More identifiers may be required according to the policy of the facility.
- Identifying the patient is a crucial step of the procedure, as improper identification may lead to potential medical errors.

3. Assembling equipment and supplies.

- Gather all the equipment and supplies required for performing the procedure.

4. Washing hands/donning PPE.

- Washing hands are performed as part of standard precautions.
- Select appropriate size gloves and don gloves.

5. Explaining procedure to the patient.

- Explaining the procedure prepares the patient for the procedure.
- The patient has the right to know about the procedure that they will be going through. Finally receive the consent from the patient for the procedure.

6. Positioning patient comfortably.

- Make sure that the patient is in a comfortable position, since some positions may compromise the procedure.

7. Checking to review if the patient is on medication or dietary restrictions.

- Check for any medication (aspirin, warfarin or heparin or others) or dietary restrictions; as some medications may increase the bleeding time.

- Follow your facility policy if the patient is on medication before the procedure is performed.
- Check if any dietary restrictions are to be followed before the procedure is performed.

PROCEDURE PHASE

SITE SELECTION

8. Selecting incision site.

- Incision site should be carefully selected.
- Site: Middle or ring finger.

Note: Follow the facility guidelines.

9. Disinfecting site with isopropyl alcohol.

- Disinfect site by appropriately cleansing the site using 70% isopropyl alcohol prep pad.
- Let the site air-dry.

10. Uncapping the reagent strip container.

  o Draw a reagent strip from the reagent strip container and insert the strip into the blood glucose device.
  o Recap the reagent strip container.

11. Positioning the device onto the selected finger.

- Perform incision perpendicular to the fingerprints using a lancet and dispose the lancet into a sharps container.

12. Placing blood onto the reagent strip.

13. Applying bandage on the incision site.

14. Reading results from the blood glucose device.

15. Cleaning the blood glucose device.

GLOVE REMOVAL, DISPOSAL AND HAND HYGIENE

16. Removing gloves using the proper technique of glove removal.

17. Disposing of gloves and other supplies into their appropriate containers.

18. Washing hands using the proper technique of hand washing.

DOCUMENTATION

19. Documenting the procedure electronically or manually.

- Follow your facility policy on documenting the procedure.

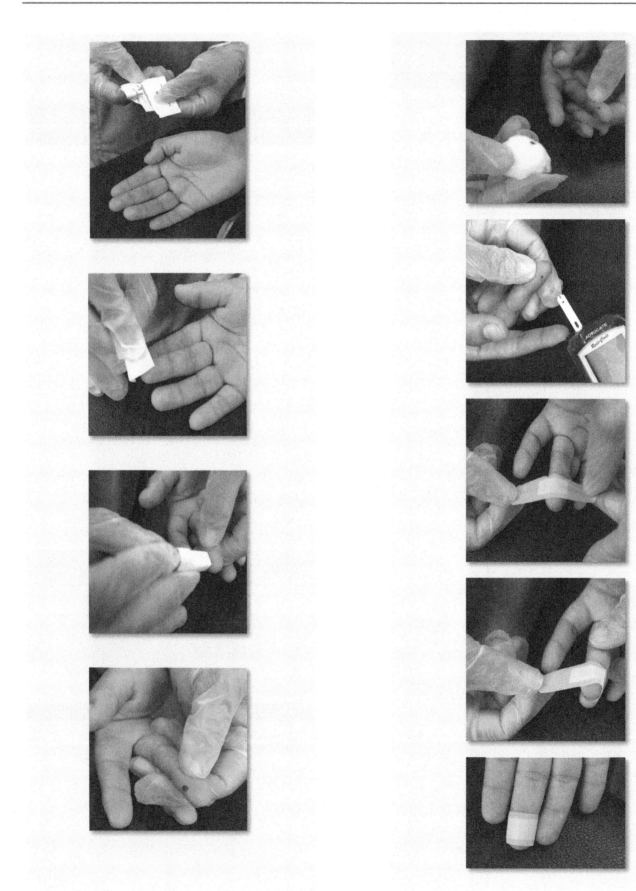

Fig 5.3 Glucose Testing

COMPETENCY CHECKLIST 5.4: CAPILLARY TUBE BLOOD COLLECTION PROCEDURE

PREPARATION PHASE

1. Verifying Physician's Order.

- Depending on the facility, the phlebotomy technician might be required to read the requisition form first before proceeding to perform the procedure.
- The requisition form provides the phlebotomy technician the information about the type of procedure that is to be performed, the patient's information and other information relevant to the procedure. Therefore, read the requisition form correctly.

2. Greeting, identifying yourself, & identifying the patient (full name & date of birth).

- Greeting your patient should be done as part of work ethics. Greet and identify yourself to the patient.
- Identify patient by asking the patient's name and date of birth. More identifiers may be required according to the policy of the facility.
- Identifying the patient is a crucial step of the procedure, as improper identification may lead to potential medical errors.

3. Assembling equipment and supplies.

- Gather all the equipment and supplies required for performing the procedure.

4. Washing hands/donning PPE.

- Washing hands are performed as part of standard precautions.
- Select appropriate size gloves and don gloves.

5. Explaining procedure to the patient.

- Explaining the procedure prepares the patient for the procedure.
- The patient has the right to know about the procedure that they will be going through. Finally receive the consent from the patient for the procedure.

6. Positioning patient comfortably.

- Make sure that the patient is in a comfortable position, since some positions may compromise the procedure.

7. Checking to review if the patient is on medication or dietary restrictions.

- Check for any medication (aspirin, warfarin or heparin or others) or dietary restrictions; as some medications may increase the bleeding time.

- Follow your facility policy if the patient is on medication before the procedure is performed.
- Check if any dietary restrictions are to be followed before the procedure is performed.

PROCEDURE PHASE

SITE SELECTION

8. Selecting incision site.

- Incision site should be carefully selected.
- Site: Middle or ring finger.

Note: Follow the facility guidelines.

9. Disinfecting site with isopropyl alcohol.

- Disinfect site by appropriately cleansing the site using 70% isopropyl alcohol prep pad.
- Let the site air-dry.

10. Positioning the device onto the selected finger.

- Perform incision perpendicular to the fingerprints using a lancet and dispose the lancet into a sharps container.

11. Wiping the first drop of blood and obtaining blood using a capillary tube.

12. Sealing of capillary tube on filling the capillary tube using a clay sealant.

13. Applying bandage on the incision site.

14. Removing gloves using the proper technique of glove removal.

15. Disposing of gloves and other supplies into their appropriate containers.

16. Washing hands using the proper technique of hand washing.

17. Documenting the procedure electronically or manually.

- Follow your facility policy on documenting the procedure.
- Follow the facility policy for handling the specimen obtained.
  - Centrifuge specimen in a hematocrit centrifuge machine or,
  - Pack the specimen as per the recommended protocol to be transported to the lab.

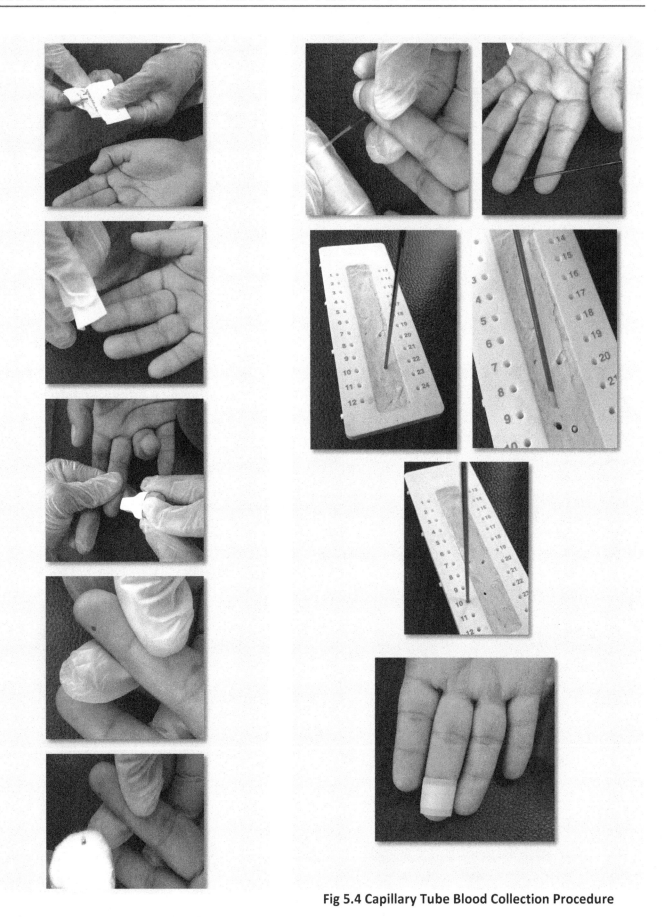

Fig 5.4 Capillary Tube Blood Collection Procedure

COMPETENCY CHECKLIST 5.5: PREPARING A BLOOD SMEAR

1. To create a blood smear, you will need two slides.
   - Sample Slide 1: Blood Sample is placed on it.
   - Slider Slide 2: Used to create a smear with a drop of blood.

2. Place the sample slide on a flat surface. Handle slides by edges only.

3. Place a tiny drop of blood near the end of the sample slide.

4. Place the end (edge) of the slider slide on the drop of the blood so that the blood spreads onto the edges of the slide.

5. Holding the slider slide at an angle of 45 degrees, push the slider slide in a forward direction creating a smear.

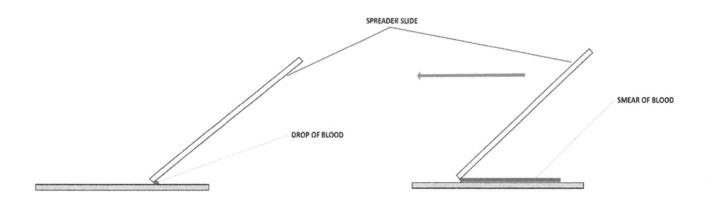

Fig 5.5 Preparing a Blood Smear

118

COMPETENCY CHECKLIST 5.6: VENIPUNCTURE USING A MULTISAMPLE NEEDLE METHOD

PREPARATION PHASE

1. Verifying Physician's Order.

- Depending on the facility, the phlebotomy technician might be required to read the requisition form first before proceeding to perform the procedure.
- The requisition form provides the phlebotomy technician the information about the type of procedure that is to be performed, the patient's information and other information relevant to the procedure. Therefore, read the requisition form correctly.

2. Greeting, identifying yourself, & identifying the patient (full name & date of birth).

- Greeting your patient should be done as part of work ethics. Greet and identify yourself to the patient.
- Identify patient by asking the patient's name and date of birth. More identifiers may be required according to the policy of the facility.
- Identifying the patient is a crucial step of the procedure, as improper identification may lead to potential medical errors.

3. Assembling equipment and supplies.

- Gather all the equipment and supplies required for performing the procedure.

4. Washing hands/donning PPE.

- Washing hands are performed as part of standard precautions.
- Select appropriate size gloves and don gloves.

5. Explaining procedure to the patient.

- Explaining the procedure prepares the patient for the procedure.
- The patient has the right to know about the procedure that they will be going through. Finally receive the consent from the patient for the procedure.
- Let the patient know that he/she will feel a small sting or pinch-like sensation when the needle is inserted into the site.

6. Positioning patient comfortably.

- Make sure that the patient is in a comfortable position, since some positions may compromise the procedure.
- The arm must be extended and oriented towards a downward position. This is done to ensure the appropriate flow of blood.

7. Checking to review if the patient is on medication or dietary restrictions.

- Check for any medication (aspirin, warfarin or heparin or others) or dietary restrictions; as some medications may increase the bleeding time.
- Follow your facility policy if the patient is on medication before the procedure is performed.
- Check if any dietary restrictions are to be followed before the procedure is performed.

PROCEDURE PHASE

TOURNIQUET APPLICATION

8. Applying tourniquet at the appropriate location.

- Should be applied correctly 3 to 4 inches proximal to the incision site.
- It should not be excessively/extremely tight or excessively/extremely loose, nor should it cause discomfort to the patient.
  - o Application if excessively/extremely tight may decrease the flow of blood to the region and also result in petechiae.
  - o Application if excessively/extremely loose may not generate enough pressure for the vein to become prominent.
- Should not be left on the patient's arm for more than 60 seconds as this can cause hemoconcentration.

SITE SELECTION

9. Selecting incision site.

- Incision site should be carefully selected. The veins available in this region for performing the procedure are:
  - o Median Cubital Vein
  - o Cephalic Vein
  - o Basilic Vein
- A palpation technique can be used to select the location of the vein.
  - o Use your finger(s) to palpate the vein by going parallel and perpendicular on the site to check for the most appropriate location.
  - o The patient may be asked to make a gentle fist.
  - o Other techniques of finding the appropriate location of the vein for the procedure may vary from facility to facility.

Note: Follow the facility guidelines for palpating and locating the vein.

10. Removing tourniquet.

- Remove the tourniquet after the site has been selected. The phlebotomy technician may also directly proceed to the next step without removing the tourniquet. It is recommended that this step is performed during training sessions or until the technique is appropriately performed. **Note: Follow the facility guidelines.**

11. Disinfecting site with isopropyl alcohol.

- Disinfect site by appropriately cleansing the site using 70% isopropyl alcohol prep pad in circles from inside to outside covering a circle diameter of 2 inches or more. Let the site air-dry.
- Do not touch the site after the site is cleansed using a 70% isopropyl alcohol prep pad. If palpation of the vein is required, you may proceed to palpate the vein and again disinfect the site.

12. Connecting needle to needle collection holder, inspect needle (use appropriate gauge needle).

- Select an appropriate gauge needle for the procedure.
- Check to see if the needle has a manufacturing defect such as
    - Damaged needle point, needle bevel or needle shaft.

13. Reapplying tourniquet.

- Should be applied correctly 3 to 4 inches proximal to the incision site.
- It should not be excessively/extremely tight or excessively/extremely loose, nor should it cause discomfort to the patient.
    - Application if excessively/extremely tight may decrease the flow of blood to the region and also result in petechiae.
    - Application if excessively/extremely loose may not generate enough pressure for the vein to become prominent.
- Should not be left on the patient's arm for more than 60 seconds as this can cause hemoconcentration.

NEEDLE INSERTION/SITE PUNCTURE

14. With the fingers (thumb or forefinger) of the non-needle unit carrying hand, pulling the skin taut below the site of the puncture.

15. With the needle unit carrying hand, inserting the needle at an appropriate angle.

- An appropriate angle must be chosen (15 degrees to 30 degrees angle)

- The bevel of the needle must face up when the needle is inserted.

16. Releasing the tourniquet when the blood starts to fill the initial tube.

- Fill the evacuated tubes in the correct order of draw.
- Release tourniquet prior to withdrawing the needle.
- Remove tourniquet within 60 seconds.

17. Removing the final tube from the evacuated tube holder prior to removing the needle.

18. Removing the needle and turning on (initiating) the safety device.

19. Applying direct pressure on incision site with a 2x2 gauze pad.

20. Disposing of sharps into a sharps container.

TUBE HANDLING AND LABELING

21. Mixing tubes (follow the correct number of inversions).

- Depending on the type of tube used, invert the tube gently and appropriately as recommended by the manufacturer or according to the facility policy.

22. Blood collection tube labeling must be performed as per the facility policy.

- Check facility policy on tube labeling.

PATIENT CARE

23. Checking on the patient for hemostasis by inspecting the site of the puncture.

24. Applying bandage once the bleeding stops.

SPECIMEN TRANSPORTATION

25. Packaging specimen for transport.

- Follow proper specimen packaging and transporting standards.

GLOVE REMOVAL, DISPOSAL AND HAND HYGIENE

26. Removing gloves using the proper technique of glove removal.

27. Disposing of gloves and other supplies into their appropriate containers.

28. Washing hands using the proper technique of hand washing.

DOCUMENTATION

29. Documenting the procedure electronically or manually.

- Follow your facility policy on documenting the procedure.

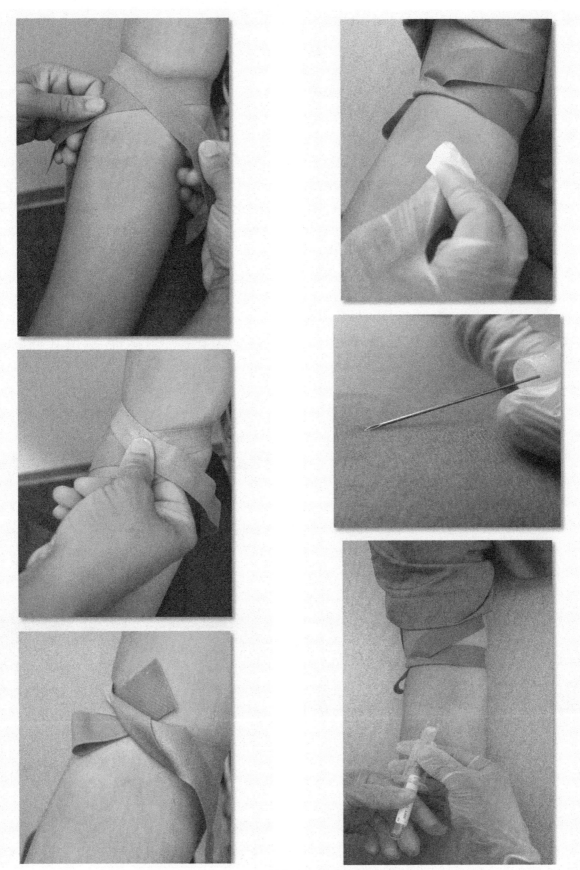

Fig 5.6 Venipuncture Using a Multisample Needle

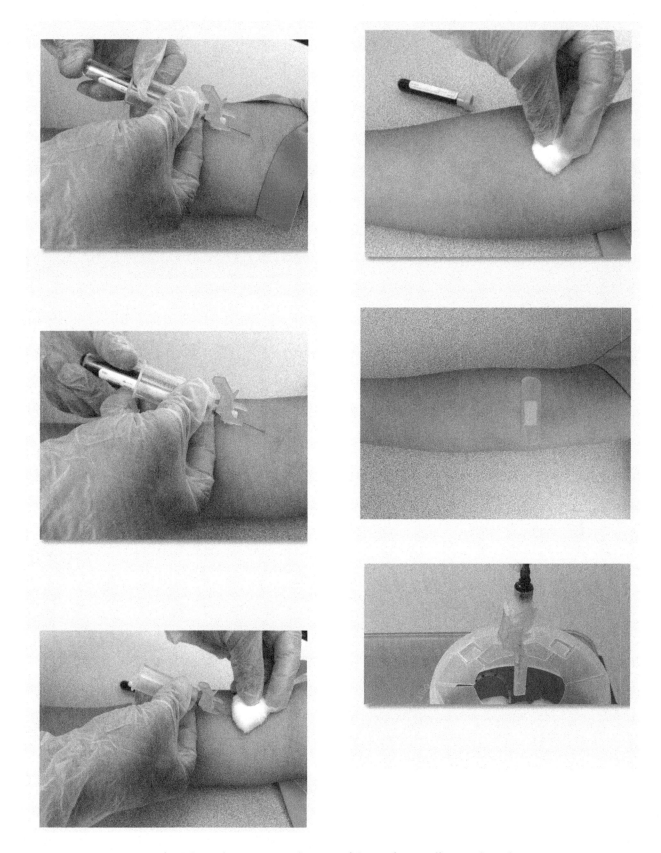

Fig 5.6 Venipuncture Using a Multisample Needle Continued

COMPETENCY CHECKLIST 5.7: VENIPUNCTURE USING A WINGED INFUSION OR BUTTERFLY NEEDLE METHOD

PREPARATION PHASE

1. Verifying Physician's Order.

- Depending on the facility, the phlebotomy technician might be required to read the requisition form first before proceeding to perform the procedure.
- The requisition form provides the phlebotomy technician the information about the type of procedure that is to be performed, the patient's information and other information relevant to the procedure. Therefore, read the requisition form correctly.

2. Greeting, identifying yourself, & identifying the patient (full name & date of birth).

- Greeting your patient should be done as part of work ethics. Greet and identify yourself to the patient.
- Identify patient by asking the patient's name and date of birth. More identifiers may be required according to the policy of the facility.
- Identifying the patient is a crucial step of the procedure, as improper identification may lead to potential medical errors.

3. Assembling equipment and supplies.

- Gather all the equipment and supplies required for performing the procedure.

4. Washing hands/donning PPE.

- Washing hands are performed as part of standard precautions.
- Select appropriate size gloves and don gloves.

5. Explaining procedure to the patient.

- Explaining the procedure prepares the patient for the procedure.
- The patient has the right to know about the procedure that they will be going through. Finally receive the consent from the patient for the procedure.
- Let the patient know that he/she will feel a small sting or pinch-like sensation when the needle is inserted into the site.

6. Positioning patient comfortably.

- Make sure that the patient is in a comfortable position, since some positions may compromise the procedure.

- The arm must be extended and oriented towards a downward position. This is done to ensure the appropriate flow of blood.

7. Checking to review if the patient is on medication or dietary restrictions.

- Check for any medication (aspirin, warfarin or heparin or others) or dietary restrictions; as some medications may increase the bleeding time.
- Follow your facility policy if the patient is on medication before the procedure is performed.
- Check if any dietary restrictions are to be followed before the procedure is performed.

PROCEDURE PHASE

TOURNIQUET APPLICATION

8. Applying tourniquet at the appropriate location.

- Should be applied correctly 2 to 3 inches proximal to the incision site.
- It should not be excessively/extremely tight or excessively/extremely loose, nor should it cause discomfort to the patient.
  a) Application if excessively/extremely tight may decrease the flow of blood to the region and also result in petechiae.
  b) Application if excessively/extremely loose may not generate enough pressure for the vein to become prominent.
- Should not be left on the patient's arm for more than 60 seconds as this can cause hemoconcentration.

SITE SELECTION

9. Selecting incision site.

- Incision site should be carefully selected. The vein available in this region for performing the procedure is:
  o Dorsal Metacarpal Vein (back of hand)
- A palpation technique can be used to select the location of the vein.
  o Use your finger(s) to palpate the vein by going parallel and perpendicular on the site to check for the most appropriate location.
- Note: Follow the facility guidelines for palpating and locating the vein.

10. Removing tourniquet.

- Remove the tourniquet after the site has been selected. The phlebotomy technician may also directly proceed to the next step without removing the tourniquet. It is recommended that this step is performed during training sessions or until the technique is appropriately performed. **Note: Follow the facility guidelines.**

11. Disinfecting site with isopropyl alcohol.

- Disinfect site by appropriately cleansing the site using 70% isopropyl alcohol prep pad in circles from inside to outside covering a circle diameter of 2 inches or more. Let the site air-dry.
- Do not touch the site after the site is cleansed using a 70% isopropyl alcohol prep pad. If palpation of the vein is required, you may proceed to palpate the vein and again disinfect the site.

12. Connecting butterfly needle to needle collection holder, inspect needle (use appropriate gauge needle).

- Select an appropriate gauge needle for the procedure.
- Check to see if the needle has a manufacturing defect such as
   a) Damaged needle point, needle bevel or needle shaft.

13. Reapplying tourniquet.

- Should be applied correctly 2 to 3 inches proximal to the incision site.
- It should not be excessively/extremely tight or excessively/extremely loose, nor should it cause discomfort to the patient.
   a) Application if excessively/extremely tight may decrease the flow of blood to the region and also result in petechiae.
   b) Application if excessively/extremely loose may not generate enough pressure for the vein to become prominent.
- Should not be left on the patient's arm for more than 60 seconds as this can cause hemoconcentration.

NEEDLE INSERTION/SITE PUNCTURE

14. With the butterfly needle unit carrying hand, inserting the needle at an appropriate angle.

- An appropriate angle must be chosen (15 degrees to 30 degrees angle)
- The bevel of the needle must face up when the needle is inserted.

15. Releasing the tourniquet when the blood starts to fill the initial tube.

- Fill the evacuated tubes in the correct order of draw.
- Release tourniquet prior to withdrawing the needle.
- Remove tourniquet within 60 seconds.

16. Removing the final tube from the evacuated tube holder prior to removing the needle.

17. Removing the needle and turning on (initiating) the safety device.

18. Applying direct pressure on incision site with a 2x2 gauze pad.

19. Disposing of sharps into a sharps container.

TUBE HANDLING AND LABELING

20. Mixing tubes (follow the correct number of inversions).

- Depending on the type of tube used, invert the tube gently and appropriately as recommended by the manufacturer or according to the facility policy.

21. Blood collection tube labeling must be performed as per the facility policy.

- Check facility policy on tube labeling.

PATIENT CARE

22. Checking on the patient for hemostasis by inspecting the site of the puncture.

23. Applying bandage once the bleeding stops.

SPECIMEN TRANSPORTATION

24. Packaging specimen for transport.

- Follow proper specimen packaging and transporting standards.

GLOVE REMOVAL, DISPOSAL AND HAND HYGIENE

25. Removing gloves using the proper technique of glove removal.

26. Disposing of gloves and other supplies into their appropriate containers.

27. Washing hands using the proper technique of hand washing.

DOCUMENTATION

28. Documenting the procedure electronically or manually.

- Follow your facility policy on documenting the procedure.

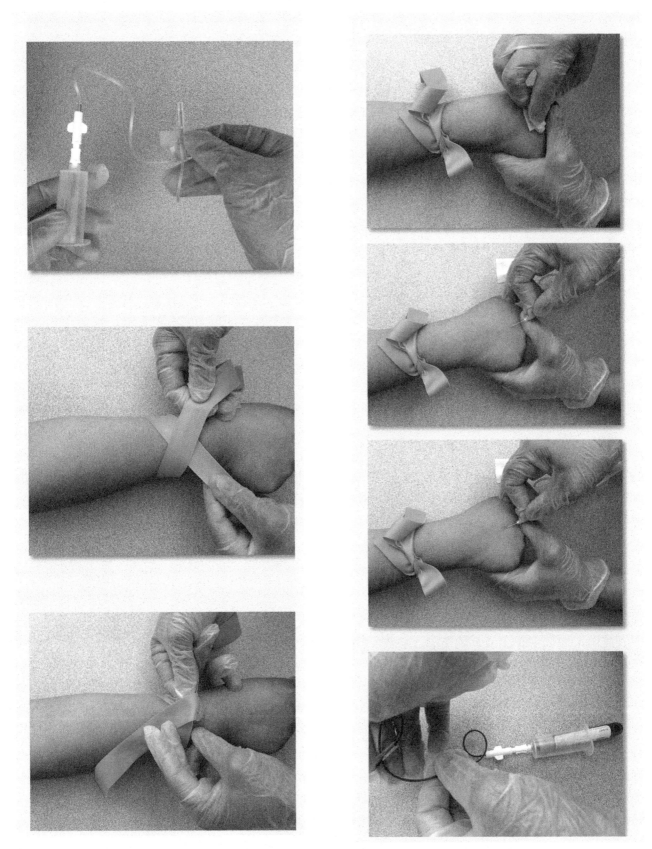

Fig 5.7 Venipuncture Using a Winged Infusion or Butterfly Needle

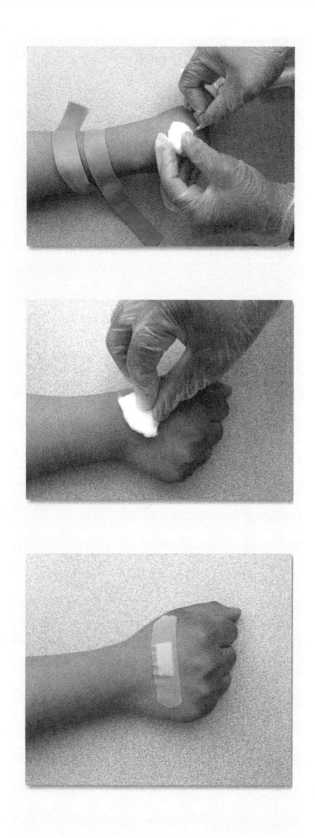

Fig 5.7 Venipuncture Using a Winged Infusion or Butterfly Needle Continued

COMPETENCY CHECKLIST 5.8: VENIPUNCTURE USING A SYRINGE AND NEEDLE (METHOD)

PREPARATION PHASE

1   Verifying Physician's Order.

- Depending on the facility, the phlebotomy technician might be required to read the requisition form first before proceeding to perform the procedure.
- The requisition form provides the phlebotomy technician the information about the type of procedure that is to be performed, the patient's information and other information relevant to the procedure. Therefore, read the requisition form correctly.

2   Greeting, identifying yourself, & identifying the patient (full name & date of birth).

- Greeting your patient should be done as part of work ethics. Greet and identify yourself to the patient.
- Identify patient by asking the patient's name and date of birth. More identifiers may be required according to the policy of the facility.
- Identifying the patient is a crucial step of the procedure, as improper identification may lead to potential medical errors.

3   Assembling equipment and supplies.

- Gather all the equipment and supplies required for performing the procedure.

4   Washing hands/donning PPE.

- Washing hands are performed as part of standard precautions.
- Select appropriate size gloves and don gloves.

5.   Explaining procedure to the patient.

- Explaining the procedure prepares the patient for the procedure.
- The patient has the right to know about the procedure that they will be going through. Finally receive the consent from the patient for the procedure.
- Let the patient know that he/she will feel a small sting or pinch-like sensation when the needle is inserted into the site.

6.   Positioning patient comfortably.

- Make sure that the patient is in a comfortable position, since some positions may compromise the procedure.
- The arm must be extended and oriented towards a downward position. This is done to ensure the appropriate flow of blood.

7.   Checking to review if the patient is on medication or dietary restrictions.

- Check for any medication (aspirin, warfarin or heparin or others) or dietary restrictions; as some medications may increase the bleeding time.
- Follow your facility policy if the patient is on medication before the procedure is performed.
- Check if any dietary restrictions are to be followed before the procedure is performed.

PROCEDURE PHASE

TOURNIQUET APPLICATION

8.   Applying tourniquet at the appropriate location.

- Should be applied correctly 3 to 4 inches proximal to the incision site.
- It should not be excessively/extremely tight or excessively/extremely loose, nor should it cause discomfort to the patient.
  - o   Application if excessively/extremely tight may decrease the flow of blood to the region and also result in petechiae.
  - o   Application if excessively/extremely loose may not generate enough pressure for the vein to become prominent.
- Should not be left on the patient's arm for more than 60 seconds as this can cause hemoconcentration.

SITE SELECTION

9.   Selecting incision site.

- Incision site should be carefully selected. The veins available in this region for performing the procedure are:
  - o   Median Cubital Vein
  - o   Cephalic Vein
  - o   Basilic Vein
- A palpation technique can be used to select the location of the vein.
  - o   Use your finger(s) to palpate the vein by going parallel and perpendicular on the site to check for the most appropriate location.
  - o   The patient may be asked to make a gentle fist.
  - o   Other techniques of finding the appropriate location of the vein for the procedure may vary from facility to facility.

Note: Follow the facility guidelines for palpating and locating the vein.

10.   Removing tourniquet.

- Remove the tourniquet after the site has been selected. The phlebotomy technician may also directly proceed to the next step without removing the tourniquet. It is recommended that this step is performed during training sessions or until the technique is appropriately performed. **Note: Follow the facility guidelines.**

11. Disinfecting site with isopropyl alcohol.

- Disinfect site by appropriately cleansing the site using 70% isopropyl alcohol prep pad in circles from inside to outside covering a circle diameter of 2 inches or more. Let the site air-dry.
- Do not touch the site after the site is cleansed using a 70% isopropyl alcohol prep pad. If palpation of the vein is required, you may proceed to palpate the vein and again disinfect the site.

12. Connecting needle to the syringe, inspecting needle (use appropriate gauge needle).

- Select an appropriate gauge needle for the procedure.
- Check to see if the needle has a manufacturing defect such as
  - Damaged needle point, needle bevel or needle shaft.
- The needle must remain capped.

13. Reapplying tourniquet.

- Should be applied correctly 3 to 4 inches proximal to the incision site.

NEEDLE INSERTION/SITE PUNCTURE

14. With the fingers (thumb or forefinger) of the non-needle-syringe unit carrying hand, pulling the skin taut below the site of the puncture.

15. With the needle-syringe unit carrying hand, inserting the needle at an appropriate angle.

- An appropriate angle must be chosen (15 degrees to 30 degrees angle)
- The bevel of the needle must face up when the needle is inserted.
- Filling the syringe by pulling the plunger of the needle backward.

16. Releasing the tourniquet.

- Release tourniquet prior to withdrawing the needle.
- Remove tourniquet within 60 seconds.

17. Removing the needle.

18. Applying direct pressure on incision site with a 2x2 gauze pad.

19. Using a transfer device. The blood from the syringe is transferred into the evacuated tube.

20. Disposing of sharps into a sharps container.

TUBE HANDLING AND LABELING

21. Mixing tube (follow the correct number of inversions).

- Depending on the type of tube used, invert the tube gently and appropriately as recommended by the manufacturer or according to the facility policy.

22. Blood collection tube labeling must be performed as per the facility policy.

- Check facility policy on tube labeling.

PATIENT CARE

23. Checking on the patient for hemostasis by inspecting the site of the puncture.

24. Applying bandage once the bleeding stops.

SPECIMEN TRANSPORTATION

25. Packaging specimen for transport.

- Follow proper specimen packaging and transporting standards.

GLOVE REMOVAL, DISPOSAL AND HAND HYGIENE

26. Removing gloves using the proper technique of glove removal.

27. Disposing of gloves and other supplies into their appropriate containers.

28. Washing hands using the proper technique of hand washing.

DOCUMENTATION

29. Documenting the procedure electronically or manually.

- Follow your facility policy on documenting the procedure.

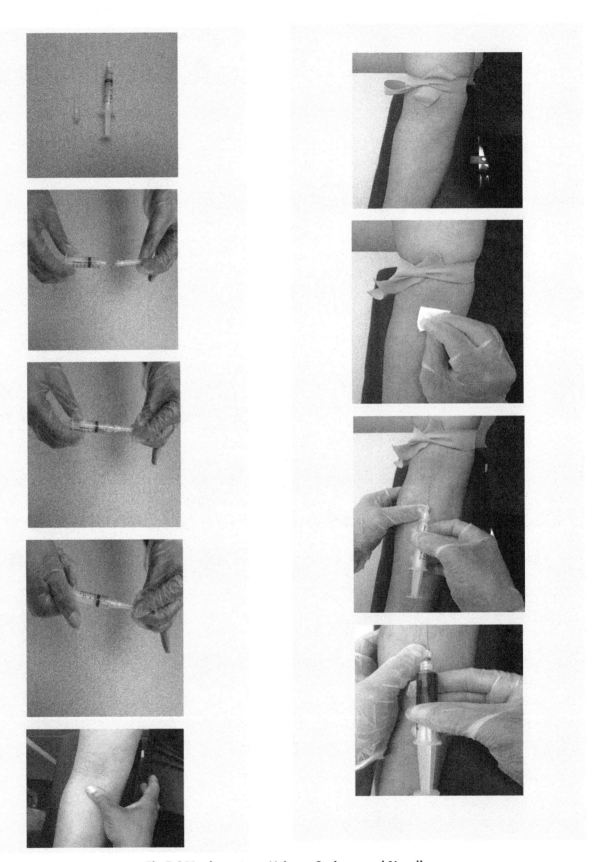

Fig 5.8 Venipuncture Using a Syringe and Needle

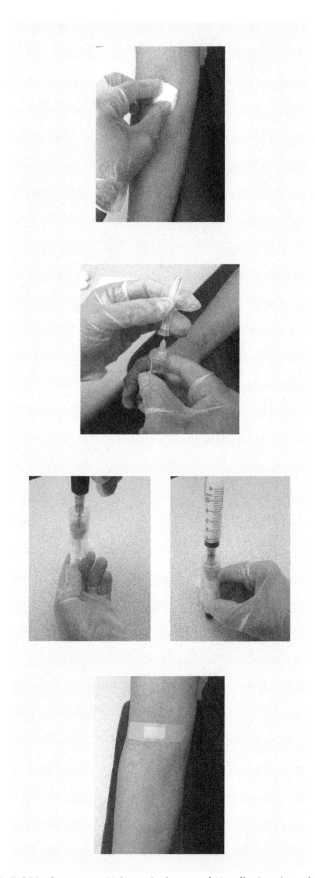

Fig 5.8 Venipuncture Using a Syringe and Needle Continued....

CHAPTER 5
END OF CHAPTER REVIEW QUESTIONS
Question Set 1: Match the following

Answers	Column A	Column B
	Inspect needle	a. To prevent medical errors
	Identify patient	b. To follow standard precautions
	Fill evacuated tubes in the correct order of draw.	c. To get consent
	Package specimen for transport	d. Procedural standard
	Verify physician's orders	e. To check for bent, clogged or broken parts
	Explain procedure to the patient	f. To prevent tissue or nerve damage
	Insert needle at an appropriate angle. (15° to 30° angle)	g. To prevent contamination
	Blot blood at 30-seconds intervals until bleeding stops	h. To prevent hemoconcentration
	Wash hands/don PPE	i. Check to see if the specimen is light, time, and temperature sensitive.
	Remove tourniquet within 60 seconds	j. To prevent misidentification

Question Set 2: ESSAY QUESTIONS

1. Explain the importance of needle insertion angle.
2. Explain in brief the advantage of using a tourniquet.
3. Why should the tourniquet be removed within 60 seconds?
4. Why is patient identification crucial for venipuncture and dermal puncture procedures?
5. Explain the procedure for preparing a blood smear.
6. List the most commonly used venipuncture sites for evacuated tube method, butterfly method, and syringe methods.
7. Explain in brief about "Explaining the procedure to the patient and getting consent.
8. Why should the needle be inspected before performing venipuncture?

Question Set 3: FILL IN THE BLANKS

1. Washing hands is performed as a part of _____, select appropriate size glove and don gloves.
2. While performing bleeding time test, blot blood with a filter paper at every _____ seconds and keep recording until the bleeding completely stops.
3. While collecting blood in the capillary tube, hold the tube _____ to avoid air bubbles during collection.
4. After collecting blood in the capillary tube, seal it with a _____ sealant.
5. While collecting blood in the capillary tube, make sure that the patient is in a comfortable position since some position may compromise the procedure. The finger used should be in a _____ position to get proper blood flow.
6. Lancet should be placed _____ to the finger prints or whorls.
7. Perform incision at the site & wipe away first drop of blood, dispose of the lancet used for incision on the site in a _____ container.

Question Set 4: MULTIPLE CHOICE QUESTIONS
CIRCLE ANSWERS

1. Lancet is used in which of the following procedures.
    a. Evacuated Tube Collection method
    b. Capillary Tube collection method
    c. Winged infusion set (venipuncture)
    d. None of the above

2. Which of the following is the correct angle at which of the needle should be inserted?
    a. 10 – 20 Degrees
    b. 15 – 30 Degrees
    c. 30 – 45 Degrees
    d. 45 – 60 Degrees

3. A reagent strip is used in which of the following procedure?
    a. Evacuated Tube Collection method
    b. Glucose testing
    c. Winged infusion set (venipuncture)
    d. None of the above

4. Which of the following is not used for venipuncture procedure?
    a. Median Cubital Vein
    b. Cephalic Vein
    c. Basilic Vein
    d. Axillary Vein

5. Which of the following procedure may require a use of transfer device?
    a. Evacuated tube collection method using needle
    b. Winged Infusion Set method using butterfly needle
    c. Syringe blood collection method using hypodermic needle
    d. Capillary tube blood collection method

6. Which of the following is not a procedural step of an evacuated tube blood collection method?
    a. Cleaning the site with isopropyl alcohol
    b. Inspecting the needle for defects
    c. Using capillary tubes for blood collection
    d. Applying tourniquet proximal to the site of venipuncture

7. Which of the following is not a procedural step of a capillary tube blood collection method?
    a. Position the device perpendicular to the fingerprints or whorls of the incision site, while holding the finger (middle or ring finger)
    b. Inspect Needle
    c. Seal the capillary tube with a clay sealant.
    d. Dispose of sharps and contaminated supplies

8. The tourniquet should be removed within_____ seconds from the time of its application.
    a. 15 seconds
    b. 30 seconds
    c. 120 seconds
    d. 60 seconds

9. Which of the following is a site used for bleeding time test procedure?
    a. Antecubital crease on the palmar surface of the forearm
    b. Median cubital vein
    c. Middle finger
    d. Ring finger

Question Set 5: TRUE OR FALSE (T/F)
CIRCLE ANSWERS

1. During the venipuncture procedure, the angle of insertion of the needle should be 30 - 45^0.
    Answer: TRUE OR FALSE

2. Lancet should be disposed of into a sharps container after the venipuncture procedure.
    Answer: TRUE OR FALSE

3. During a bleeding time test, the blood should be wicked or wiped every 60 seconds.
    Answer: TRUE OR FALSE

4. During capillary tube blood collection method, the incision should be made parallel to the finger whorls.
    Answer: TRUE OR FALSE

5. Always explain the procedure to the patient prior to performing the procedure.
    Answer: TRUE OR FALSE

6. The blood pressure cuff should be inflated to 80mmhg while performing the bleeding time test.

Answer: TRUE OR FALSE

7. Middle finger or ring finger are incision sites used for dermal puncture procedure.
   Answer: TRUE OR FALSE

8. Location-appropriate for applying tourniquet should be 3 to 4 inches proximal to the incision site (antecubital region).
   Answer: TRUE OR FALSE

9. Identifying the patient is a crucial step of the procedure as improper identification can lead to potential medical errors.
   Answer: TRUE OR FALSE

10. Disinfecting incision site should be done by cleaning the site with 70 % isopropyl alcohol (concentric circles from inside to outside).
    Answer: TRUE OR FALSE

Question Set 6: Clinical Competency Checklist Critical Thinking (CT):
Fill in the correct abbreviations rationale for the steps enlisted in each procedure.

PS	Procedural Standard
SP	Standard Precaution
PME	Prevent Medical Error
AC	Avoid Complication
WE	Work Ethics
TRANS	Transportation
PBR	Patients' Bill Of Rights
DOCU	Documentation

COMPETENCY CHECKLIST 5.2: BLEEDING TIME COMPETENCY	CRITICAL THINKING
1. Verifying Physician's Order.	
2. Greeting, identifying yourself, & identifying the patient (full name & date of birth).	
3. Assembling equipment and supplies.	
4. Washing hands/donning PPE.	
5. Explaining procedure to the patient.	
6. Positioning patient comfortably.	

7. Checking to review if the patient is on medication or dietary restrictions.	
8. Selecting incision site.	
9. Disinfecting site with isopropyl alcohol.	
10. Applying blood pressure cuff.	
11. Positioning the device onto the palmar surface of the forearm.	
12. Blotting blood at 30-second intervals until bleeding stops.	
13. Removing blood pressure cuff.	
14. Applying bandage on the incision site.	
15. Disposing of sharps into a sharps container.	
16. Removing gloves using the proper technique of glove removal.	
17. Disposing of gloves and other supplies into their appropriate containers.	
18. Washing hands using the proper technique of hand washing.	
19. Documenting the procedure electronically or manually.	

COMPETENCY CHECKLIST 5.3: GLUCOSE TESTING COMPETENCY	CRITICAL THINKING
1. Verifying Physician's Order.	
2. Greeting, identifying yourself, & identifying the patient (full name & date of birth).	
3. Assembling equipment and supplies.	
4. Washing hands/donning PPE.	
5. Explaining procedure to the patient.	
6. Positioning patient comfortably.	
7. Checking to review if the patient is on medication or dietary restrictions.	
8. Selecting incision site.	
9. Disinfecting site with isopropyl alcohol.	
10. Uncapping the reagent strip container.	

11. Positioning the device onto the selected finger.	
12. Placing blood onto the reagent strip.	
13. Applying bandage on the incision site.	
14. Reading results from the blood glucose device.	
15. Cleaning the blood glucose device.	
16. Removing gloves using the proper technique of glove removal.	
17. Disposing of gloves and other supplies into their appropriate containers.	
18. Washing hands using the proper technique of hand washing.	
19. Documenting the procedure electronically or manually.	

COMPETENCY CHECKLIST 5.4: CAPILLARY TUBE BLOOD COLLECTION PROCEDURE	CRITICAL THINKING
1. Verifying Physician's Order.	
2. Greeting, identifying yourself, & identifying the patient (full name & date of birth).	
3. Assembling equipment and supplies.	
4. Washing hands/donning PPE.	
5. Explaining procedure to the patient.	
6. Positioning patient comfortably.	
7. Checking to review if the patient is on medication or dietary restrictions.	
8. Selecting incision site.	
9. Disinfecting site with isopropyl alcohol.	
10. Positioning the device onto the selected finger.	
11. Wiping the first drop of blood and obtaining blood using a capillary tube.	
12. Sealing of capillary tube on filling the capillary tube using a clay sealant.	
13. Applying bandage on the incision site.	

14. Removing gloves using the proper technique of glove removal.	
15. Disposing of gloves and other supplies into their appropriate containers.	
16. Washing hands using the proper technique of hand washing.	
17. Documenting the procedure electronically or manually.	

COMPETENCY CHECKLIST 5.5: BLOOD SMEAR	CRITICAL THINKING
1. To create a blood smear, you will need two slides.	
• Sample Slide 1: Blood Sample is placed on it.	
• Slider Slide 2: Used to create a smear with a drop of blood.	
2. Place the sample slide on a flat surface. Handle slides by edges only.	
3. Place a tiny drop of blood near the end of the sample slide.	
4. Place the end (edge) of the slider slide on the drop of the blood so that the blood spreads onto the edges of the slide.	
5. Holding the slider slide at an angle of 45 degrees, push the slider slide in a forward direction creating a smear.	

COMPETENCY CHECKLIST 5.6: VENIPUNCTURE USING A MULTISAMPLE NEEDLE METHOD	CRITICAL THINKING
1. Verifying Physician's Order.	
2. Greeting, identifying yourself, & identifying the patient (full name & date of birth).	
3. Assembling equipment and supplies.	
4. Washing hands/donning PPE.	
5. Explaining procedure to the patient.	
6. Positioning patient comfortably.	
7. Checking to review if the patient is on medication or dietary restrictions.	

8. Applying tourniquet at the appropriate location.	
9. Selecting incision site.	
10. Removing tourniquet.	
11. Disinfecting site with isopropyl alcohol.	
12. Connecting needle to needle collection holder, inspect needle (use appropriate gauge needle).	
13. Reapplying tourniquet.	
14. With the fingers (thumb or forefinger) of the non-needle unit carrying hand, pulling the skin taut below the site of the puncture.	
15. With the needle unit carrying hand, inserting the needle at an appropriate angle.	
16. Releasing the tourniquet when the blood starts to fill the initial tube.	
17. Removing the final tube from the evacuated tube holder prior to removing the needle.	
18. Removing the needle and turning on (initiating) the safety device.	
19. Applying direct pressure on incision site with a 2x2 gauze pad.	
20. Disposing of sharps into a sharps container.	
21. Mixing tubes (follow the correct number of inversions).	
22. Blood collection tube labeling must be performed as per the facility policy.	
23. Checking on the patient for hemostasis by inspecting the site of the puncture.	
24. Applying bandage once the bleeding stops.	
25. Packaging specimen for transport.	
26. Removing gloves using the proper technique of glove removal.	
27. Disposing of gloves and other supplies into their appropriate containers.	
28. Washing hands using the proper technique of hand washing.	

29. Documenting the procedure electronically or manually.	
COMPETENCY CHECKLIST 5.7: VENIPUNCTURE USING A WINGED INFUSION OR BUTTERFLY NEEDLE METHOD	**CRITICAL THINKING**
1. Verifying Physician's Order.	
2. Greeting, identifying yourself, & identifying the patient (full name & date of birth).	
3. Assembling equipment and supplies.	
4. Washing hands/donning PPE.	
5. Explaining procedure to the patient.	
6. Positioning patient comfortably.	
7. Checking to review if the patient is on medication or dietary restrictions.	
8. Applying tourniquet at the appropriate location.	
9. Selecting incision site.	
10. Removing tourniquet.	
11. Disinfecting site with isopropyl alcohol.	
12. Connecting butterfly needle to needle collection holder, inspect needle (use appropriate gauge needle).	
13. Reapplying tourniquet.	
14. With the butterfly needle unit carrying hand, inserting the needle at an appropriate angle.	
15. Releasing the tourniquet when the blood starts to fill the initial tube.	
16. Removing the final tube from the evacuated tube holder prior to removing the needle.	
17. Removing the needle and turning on (initiating) the safety device.	
18. Applying direct pressure on incision site with a 2x2 gauze pad.	
19. Disposing of sharps into a sharps container.	
20. Mixing tubes (follow the correct number of inversions).	

21.	Blood collection tube labeling must be performed as per the facility policy.	
22.	Checking on the patient for hemostasis by inspecting the site of the puncture.	
23.	Applying bandage once the bleeding stops.	
24.	Packaging specimen for transport.	
25.	Removing gloves using the proper technique of glove removal.	
26.	Disposing of gloves and other supplies into their appropriate containers.	
27.	Washing hands using the proper technique of hand washing.	
28.	Documenting the procedure electronically or manually.	

COMPETENCY CHECKLIST 5.8: VENIPUNCTURE USING A SYRINGE AND NEEDLE (METHOD)	CRITICAL THINKING	
1	Verifying Physician's Order.	
2	Greeting, identifying yourself, & identifying the patient (full name & date of birth).	
3	Assembling equipment and supplies.	
4	Washing hands/donning PPE.	
5.	Explaining procedure to the patient.	
6.	Positioning patient comfortably.	
7.	Checking to review if the patient is on medication or dietary restrictions.	
8.	Applying tourniquet at the appropriate location.	
9.	Selecting incision site.	
10.	Removing tourniquet.	
11.	Disinfecting site with isopropyl alcohol.	
12.	Connecting needle to the syringe, inspecting needle (use appropriate gauge needle).	
13.	Reapplying tourniquet.	

14.	With the fingers (thumb or forefinger) of the non-needle-syringe unit carrying hand, pulling the skin taut below the site of the puncture.	
15.	With the needle-syringe unit carrying hand, inserting the needle at an appropriate angle.	
16.	Releasing the tourniquet.	
17.	Removing the needle.	
18.	Applying direct pressure on incision site with a 2x2 gauze pad.	
19.	Using a transfer device. The blood from the syringe is transferred into the evacuated tube.	
20.	Disposing of sharps into a sharps container.	
21.	Mixing tube (follow the correct number of inversions).	
22.	Blood collection tube labeling must be performed as per the facility policy.	
23.	Checking on the patient for hemostasis by inspecting the site of the puncture.	
24.	Applying bandage once the bleeding stops.	
25.	Packaging specimen for transport.	
26.	Removing gloves using the proper technique of glove removal.	
27.	Disposing of gloves and other supplies into their appropriate containers.	
28.	Washing hands using the proper technique of hand washing.	
29.	Documenting the procedure electronically or manually.	

CHAPTER 6: PHLEBOTOMY FUNDAMENTAL ESSENTIALS

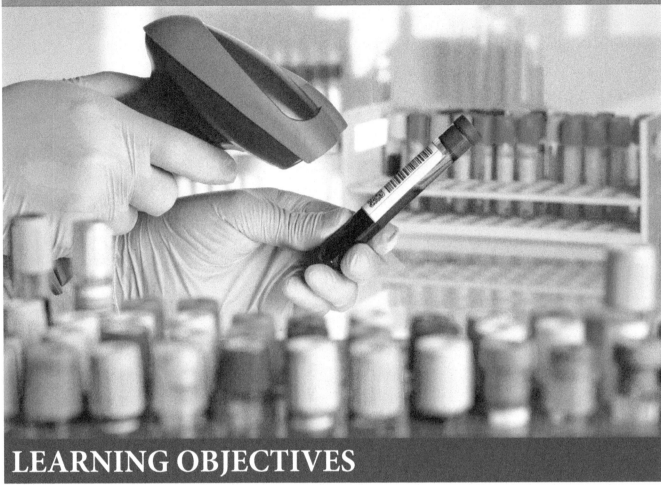

LEARNING OBJECTIVES

At the end of this chapter the student will be able to describe in brief:

- Venipuncture complications
- Areas of concern
- Tourniquet test
- How to avoid hemolysis
- Specimen labelling
- Specimen handling (light, time & temperature)
- Specimen transporting
- Precautions to be considered
- Rejection of Specimen
- Test requisition
- Other procedures

- Blood Collection from Pediatric and Neonates
- Blood Sugar Tests
- Blood Cultures
- Blood Collection for Legal Purposes
- Therapeutic Drug Monitoring (TDM)
- Urine Specimen Collection
- Stool Specimen Collection
- Sputum Specimen Collection
- Throat Swab Specimen Collection
- Blood Donation Procedure
- Safety data sheets
- Incident report

VENIPUNCTURE COMPLICATIONS

1. **Petechiae:** small spot on the skin, red or purple in color, caused by hemorrhage to the capillary (blood vessel).

2. **Arterial puncture:** this can occur as a result of hitting an artery while performing venipuncture. The blood collected in the blood collection tube as a result of an arterial puncture would be pulsating and bright red in color. If this occurs, post-procedure apply pressure to the area for 5 – 10 minutes or until bleeding has completely stopped. Check your facility policy on unintentional arterial punctures.

3. **Collapsed vein:** Internal swelling of the vein due to repeated injury causes the vein to block temporarily leading to a collapsed vein. Another reason could be the vacuum in the blood collection tube may cause the vein to collapse, this may occur due to the size of the vein or other factors.

4. **Excessive bleeding:** After the procedure, there may be excessive bleeding, it may be as a result of an improper technique or due to the patient having a condition that inhibits the clotting process (hemophilia).

5. **Uncooperative patient:** It might sometimes be difficult to draw blood from infants and children or patients that are mentally not stable.

6. **Septicemia:** Not following the precautions and proper procedural standards such as using contaminated equipment and supplies may cause infection in the blood.

7. **Thrombus:** Injury to a blood vessel leads to clot formation. This clot formation obstructs the blood flow through the blood vessel, the clot formed is known as a thrombus. The process through which it forms is known as THROMBOSIS. When this thrombus is dislodged from its location in the blood vessel, it is called an embolus, a free-floating clot. This embolus can lodge into a vessel causing a serious problem, such as infarction in the heart or stroke in the brain.

8. **Thrombophlebitis:** A blood clot formed within the vein further cause's inflammation, redness, and pain. The most common affected veins are the veins that are located closer to the surface of the skin.

9. **Pain:** Improper handling of the needle during the procedure may cause injury to the skin and the underlying structures resulting in pain.

10. **Allergic Response:** An allergic response may initiate as a result of an equipment or supply used during the procedure. The most common supply that may initiate an allergic response would be using the latex gloves.

11. **Phlebitis:** Inflammation of vein may occur due to injury to that vein due to venipuncture or due to blood clot formation. (Itis = Inflammation)

12. **Syncope (fainting):** A patient may faint (before, during or after the procedure). In such events, make sure to untie the tourniquet and withdraw the needle. Next, report the incident in an incident report as per the facility policy. Follow your facility policy in such events.

13. **Nerve Involvement:** While performing phlebotomy, if a needle hits the nerve, it may cause partial or complete damage to the nerve. The symptoms would be sharp, tingling pain. Some causes of a nerve injury during phlebotomy may include, incorrect needle angle, incorrect amount of pressure applied while performing venipuncture (phlebotomy). Phlebotomy technicians must always focus on the procedure they will be performing since a nerve damage may result in permanent damage to the patient.

14. **Seizures:** A patient may undergo seizures while the procedure is being performed. If it does, untie the tourniquet and withdraw the needle. Next, remove all articles and objects from the nearby vicinity that may injure the patient. Next, report the incident in an incident report as per the facility policy. Follow your facility policy in such events.

15. **Hematoma:** Occurs due to injury caused by the needle insertion leading to accumulation of blood external to the blood vessels and within the tissue causing internal bleeding of the tissue. Hematoma may also result from not removing the tourniquet before the needle is withdrawn or not applying appropriate pressure after the needle is withdrawn from the puncture site.

16. **Hemolysis:** A breakdown of red blood cells. Breakdown of RBCs causes the release of hemoglobin. Few causes of hemolysis are incorrect needle gauge, shaking blood collection tubes vigorously, prolong application of a tourniquet, improper site selection, improper storage of the specimen collected, and inappropriate transport procedures.

17. **Hemoconcentration:** Increase in concentration of red blood cells and other formed elements.

18. **Vasovagal reaction:** A patient may experience this as a result of a shock or pain, it can lead to fainting.

19. **Bone infection:** While performing phlebotomy, if a bone is hit with either a needle or a lancet, it may cause bone infection and inflammation.

20. **Inability to Draw Blood:** A phlebotomist may not be able to draw blood from a patient on the 1st attempt. If so, follow your facility policy on how to proceed. Some facilities may allow the second draw. However, it is best to double check your facility policy.

21. **Compartmental syndrome:** This can occur as a result of excessive bleeding post-phlebotomy procedure. Compartment syndrome occurs when more than normal pressure develops in a particular space within the human body (compartment). This excessive bleeding may result in a buildup of high pressure within the space, which further compresses the underlying structures such as the blood vessels, nerves, and other tissues. This compression (compartment syndrome) can be a medical emergency and if not treated may result in permanent damage.

Few reasons that can cause compartment syndrome post-phlebotomy:

- A patient on anticoagulants.

- A patient is suffering from a blood clotting disorder such as hemophilia.

Few steps to avoid the above mentioned:

- **Follow your facility policy and recommended guidelines.**
  - o Always ask the patient if they are on a blood thinner or anticoagulants or any other medications.
  - o Always ask the patient if he or she has a condition that inhibits the clotting of blood.

- **If venipuncture is performed on a patient on an anticoagulant.**
  - o To avoid excessive bleeding, pressure is applied on the site for prolong duration until the bleeding stops.
  - o Remember: if the bleeding does not stop, seek medical attention immediately.

AREAS OF CONCERNS

Apart from the complications of venipuncture, the phlebotomy technician must also be aware about some of the factors that may related to the:

POINTS TO CONSIDER
PROCEDURE:

1. **Procedural Steps:** Not following proper steps in performing the procedure may lead to inability to obtain blood.

2. **Vein Related Issues**
   a. Identifying the vein: Not identifying the vein appropriately may lead to inability to obtain blood.
   b. Selecting a vein that is not suitable for obtaining blood.

3. **Patient & Patient Position:** Both, the patient and the phlebotomy technician must be in a comfortable and appropriate position.

POINTS TO CONSIDER
TUBE:

1. **Tube Expiration:** Using a tube that has already expired must not be used for the procedure.

2. **Tube Condition:** Using a tube that may have been damaged.

3. **Tube Additives:** Using an incorrect tube for blood collection or the tube is not appropriately filled.

4. **Tube Position:** Not appropriately fitting the tube into the needle. Note: the tube must be gently pushed into the needle unit holder. The rear needle of a multisample needle must pierce the rubber top portion for the blood to flow into the tube.

POINTS TO CONSIDER
PUNCTURE SITE:

1. **Hematomas**
   a. Avoid sites that have a hematoma.
2. **Fistula or Cannula**
   a. Check your facility guidelines on the presence of a fistula or cannula.

b. Blood must not be drawn from these sites without proper authorization from the physician.

3. **Artery**
   a. When performing the venipuncture procedure, care must be taken to avoid puncturing an artery.

4. **Burns, Injured Area and Extensive Scarring**
   a. Avoid drawing blood from such areas.

5. **Open wound, skin sutures and recent skin conditions**
   a. Do not attempt to draw blood from areas like an open wound, skin condition, and recent sutures.

6. **Occluded Veins**
   a. Due to occlusion in the lumen of the vein, there is reduced blood flow through these veins.
   b. Obtaining blood specimen from such veins must be avoided.

7. **Obesity**
   a. Locating a vein in such events may be difficult. Using a blood pressure cuff may assist in finding the vein. Check your facility guidelines on how much inflation pressure should be applied to the patient's arm for locating the vein. Usually, the pressure inflated should not go beyond the diastolic blood pressure of the patient. The application time must be followed as per the facility guidelines.

8. **Mastectomy**
   a. Avoid taking samples from these areas. It is important to consult the physician in such cases and check with the facility guidelines.
   b. If single mastectomy, the opposite side arm may be used to draw blood.
   c. If double mastectomy, consult with the physician and follow recommended protocols.
   d. Ensure that you have proper permission (after consulting with the physician) to perform a blood draw from a mastectomy patient.

9. **IV Site**
   a. Such site must be avoided.
   b. However, if no other site is available. The phlebotomy technician must request that the IV line is turned off for 2 minutes. **Only a**

trained staff must turn off the line. The phlebotomy technician **must not** try and turn off the IV line. Blood Draw must be from a site below the IV Site. Also, the application of the tourniquet must be in between the IV Site and the puncture site. While documenting the procedure, it must be documented that the blood draw was performed from a site below (proximal) the IV Site. **Follow your facility guidelines in such situations.**

10. **Edematous Extremities**
    a. Avoid taking a specimen from such sites as the specimens collected from these sites are contaminated with other tissue fluids. Moreover, it may be difficult to find the vein from such sites due to the presence of swelling.

POINTS TO CONSIDER
NEEDLE POSITION:

1. Needle insertion angle is more than 30 degrees.

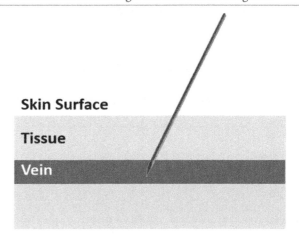

2. Needle insertion angle is less than 15 degrees.

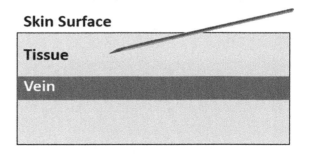

3. The needle did not penetrate into a vein.

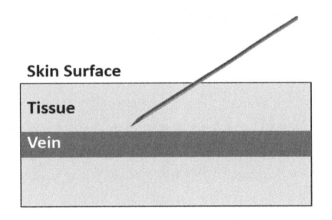

6. Collapsed vein (proper angle but vein collapsed)

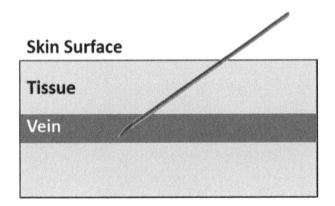

4. The needle penetrates too far into a vein.

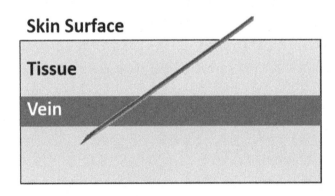

7. The needle is in the vein at 15 to 30 Degree.

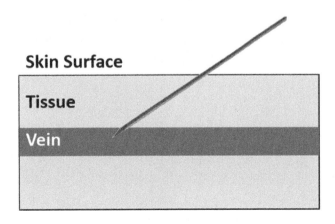

5. The needle just penetrated the wall but is not in the vein.

PATIENT:

1. **Identification issue:** The phlebotomy technician may not correctly identify the patient as per the standard procedure guidelines.

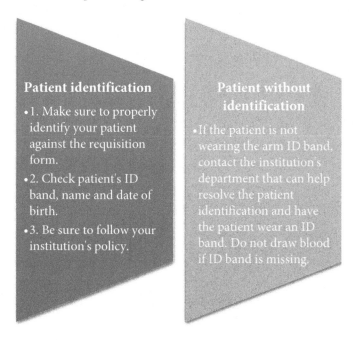

Patient identification

- 1. Make sure to properly identify your patient against the requisition form.
- 2. Check patient's ID band, name and date of birth.
- 3. Be sure to follow your institution's policy.

Patient without identification

- If the patient is not wearing the arm ID band, contact the institution's department that can help resolve the patient identification and have the patient wear an ID band. Do not draw blood if ID band is missing.

2. **Co-operation issue:** The patient may not co-operate with the phlebotomy technician.

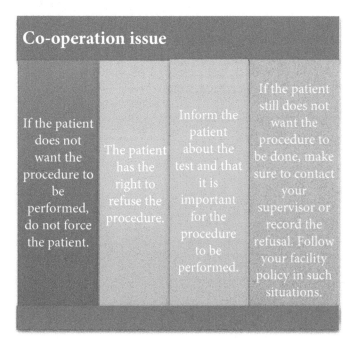

Co-operation issue

If the patient does not want the procedure to be performed, do not force the patient.

The patient has the right to refuse the procedure.

Inform the patient about the test and that it is important for the procedure to be performed.

If the patient still does not want the procedure to be done, make sure to contact your supervisor or record the refusal. Follow your facility policy in such situations.

3. **Interaction issue:** The phlebotomy technician may not be able to complete the procedure if the patient does not understand the language.

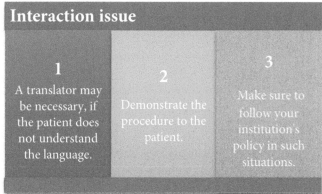

Interaction issue

1 A translator may be necessary, if the patient does not understand the language.

2 Demonstrate the procedure to the patient.

3 Make sure to follow your institution's policy in such situations.

Remember "iCi" i: Identification C: Co-operation i: Interaction.

TOURNIQUET:

- **Improper application technique:** Not being able to tie the tourniquet appropriately on the patient's arm.
- **Excessive Pressure:** Application of the tourniquet is excessively tight on the patient's arm.
- **Insufficient Pressure:** Application of the tourniquet is excessively loose on the patient's arm, therefore it is unable to create sufficient pressure.
- **Improper application location:** Application of the tourniquet is NOT in the correct location on the patient's arm.

Note: Follow proper technique in order to tie the tourniquet onto the patient's arm.

TOURNIQUET TEST

This test is done to check the capillary fragility. To start this test, you will need to apply blood pressure cuff on the patient's arm. The blood pressure cuff must be inflated between systolic and diastolic blood pressure for a recommended duration. Next, remove the blood pressure cuff and check for the number of Petechiae within the 5 cm circle.

Normal	If less than 15 Petechiae.
Fragile Capillaries	If more than 15 Petechiae are seen.

DISINFECTION:

Disinfecting the site of puncture is an integral step of performing the (venipuncture or dermal puncture) procedure. Post cleaning the site, allow the site to air dry.

1. If **70% isopropyl alcohol** is not the recommended antiseptic that can be used for the procedure, use:

    a. **Povidone Iodine (water based)**

        i.   If doing a dermal puncture, do not use povidone iodine.

        ii. For blood culture specimen collection, use povidone iodine.

2. If **70% isopropyl alcohol and povidone iodine** are not the recommended antiseptic for the procedure, use

    a. **Chlorhexidine Gluconate (2%)**

3. If the test is being performed for "LEGAL BLOOD ALCOHOL LEVEL" do not use alcohol for cleaning the site.

Note: Follow your facility policy on recommended uses of antiseptic solution, wipes, swabs, etc. for cleaning the site according to the procedure to be performed to draw blood specimens.

HOW TO AVOID HEMOLYSIS?

a. **Improper inversion technique in order to mix the blood and additive after the blood is collected into the evacuated tube.**

    The correct technique is to gently invert the tube for the recommended times.

b. **Under-filling of the tube with additives may result in hemolysis.**

    To avoid this, the tube must be filled appropriately (blood to additive ratio). The vacuum in the tube will allow the tube to fill with blood.

c. **Avoid drawing blood from an area that has a hematoma.**

    To avoid specimen contamination, areas that have hematoma must be avoided.

d. **Never instruct the patient to pump their fist.**

    This must be avoided. The patient must be instructed to make a gentle fist.

e. **Select the correct size needle.**

The size of the needle selected must be appropriate to the patient's vein.

f. **Exposing the specimen to extreme temperatures post collection.**

    Do not leave the specimen to expose to extreme temperatures, follow your facility policy on storing the collected specimens.

g. **Improper handling of the specimens while transporting.**

    Be careful while transporting the specimen, not handling the specimens properly may cause the specimen to undergo hemolysis.

h. **Puncture site wet with alcohol.**

    The puncture site must air-dry before the puncture is performed.

SPECIMEN LABELING

Specimen labeling is of two types:

MANUAL LABEL	By writing the required information onto a label and appropriately applying it onto the tube.
COMPUTER GENERATED LABEL	Required information is already available on the label. The only information that may be required to be added would be the time and date of the draw along with the initials and or name of the phlebotomy technician collecting the specimen.

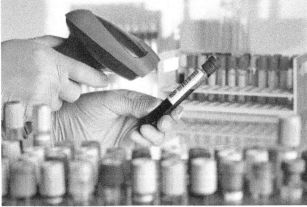

Scanning barcode on blood collection tube

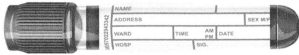

Sample label on blood collection tube.

GENERAL INFORMATION REQUIRED:

Patient must be appropriately identified, and such information should be available before and/or at the time of labeling the specimen.

1. The specimen must contain the patient information (e.g. first and last name, date of birth and or medical record number of the patient, etc.).

2. The specimen must contain the date on which the specimen is being collected.

3. The specimen must contain the time on which the specimen is being collected.

4. The specimen must contain the name and initials of the person that collected the specimen (see institution policy).

5. The label must be appropriately placed onto the tube(s).

Follow your facility policy on specimen labeling and the required information that must be available on the specimen tube.

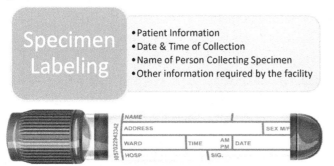

Figure 6.1 Labeled Specimen

SPECIMEN HANDLING

After collection of specimen, care should be taken to handle the specimen properly as improper handling may lead to change in composition of the collected specimen due to external factors like:

- Exposure to Light
- Time
- Temperature

– Make sure to invert tube as per the recommended guidelines. Inverting tubes inappropriately may lead to improper mixing of the additive and the specimen collected. Do not vigorously shake the tube.

– Make sure to label the specimen correctly.

– Make sure that every specimen collected is packaged in a leak proof and closed container.

LIGHT SENSITIVE SPECIMENS

1. Some specimens may be light sensitive, which means, if the specimen is exposed to light, the specimen may change its composition. Therefore these specimens must be protected from light during their storage & transport.

2. Few tests that require the specimen to be protected from light are: bilirubin, biotin, porphyrin, carotene, vitamin A, vitamin B1, B2, B3, B6, E and K.

3. Cover the tube with foil or an opaque bag or with an amber plastic tube.

4. Follow your institution policy on protecting light-sensitive specimens.

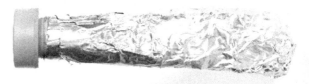

Figure 6.2 Light Sensitive Specimen

TIME SENSITIVE SPECIMENS

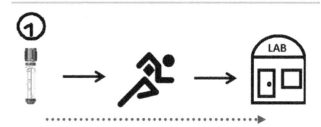

Figure 6.3 Time Sensitive Specimen Transport

Time Sensitive Specimen

Some tube specimens are time sensitive which means that with time the composition of the specimen may change. It is important to transport specimens to the laboratory as quickly as possible after collecting them.

STAT Tests

Results of the STAT (immediate) test are required on a priority basis. It is needed for diagnosis or providing treatment. The laboratory receiving a **STAT** specimen gives such specimen a high priority. The packaging of the specimen must display that the specimen is a 'STAT' specimen.

TYPES OF TEST REQUEST	
STAT	Requires immediate test results.
ASAP	Requires test results as soon as possible but not immediately.
ROUTINE	Requires test results (not immediately or as soon as possible).
TIMED	A blood draw is performed at a specific time, and test results are reported as routine. If required as a STAT order, the results are required immediately.

REMEMBER SART: STAT, ASAP, ROUTINE, TIMED.

Follow your institution's tests and result reporting guidelines.

TEMPERATURE SENSITIVE SPECIMENS

Some specimens are temperature sensitive, which means that if the specimen is not protected from temperature, it may lead to a change in the composition of the specimen.

1) **Specimens that require warm temperature:** Specimens that require the specimen be kept in a warm temperature must be done by placing the specimen at a recommended temperature. Specimens such as cold agglutinins (Collect specimen in a pre-warm recommended tube and place the specimen in 37 degrees C incubator, the temperature must be maintained until the serum is separated from the specimen), cryoglobulin, cryofibrinogen.

   E.g. Use of warm bath or incubator or heat packs.

2) **Specimens that require cold temperature.**
   Specimens that require the specimen be kept in a cold temperature must be done by placing the specimen at a recommended temperature.

   E.g. Use of ice.

   Follow your facility guidelines on the type of product to be used to keep the specimen warm or cold.

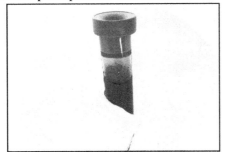

Figure 6.4a

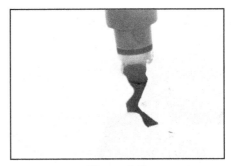

Figure 6.4b
Chilled Specimen

SPECIMEN TRANSPORTING

The specimen collected and packed must be transported to the proper facility. The facility in most cases would be the laboratory.

Transporting within the institution:

There are several ways to transport specimen within the institution

1. By either delivering the specimen to the required location or
2. By use of a pneumatic tube system (only if recommended).

Transporting from institution to the laboratory:

There are 2 ways in which the specimen can reach the laboratory.

1. By either delivering the specimen to the laboratory or
2. By contacting the laboratory for a pickup.

Note: always follow the facility guidelines on transporting the specimen.

-   Make sure to keep the specimen tubes in a vertical position for transportation.
-   Specimens must have a biohazard label on the packing.
-   Specimens must be transported to the laboratory for analysis at the earliest.
-   Specimens are usually transported at room temperature unless a chilling specimen is recommended.
-   Local, state and national standards and regulations as applicable must be followed while transporting specimens.

ABSENCE & MIXING OF ADDITIVES

1. **Absence of additive**
   This may occur if the blood & additive from the blood collection tube flows back into the vein from which the blood is being collected, this will result in reduced levels of additive left in the tube for the specimen collected, which may lead to an inappropriate proportion of additive to the specimen collected.

2. **Mixing of Additives**
   As mentioned above (**absence of additive**), that the blood & additive from the tube may flow back into the vein. If drawing multiple samples, there will be mixing of additive from earlier tube to the later tube since the same blood with the additive in the patient's vein may now be collected into the later tube.

   How can this be prevented?

   - **The position of the patient's arm:** must be in a downward position.
   - **The position of the blood collection tube:** must be held in such a position that the blood being collected and the additive present in the tube do not flow back into the vein.

PRECAUTIONS TO BE CONSIDERED

BLOOD VOLUME

Drawing **INCREASED** amount of blood than recommended for an individual may lead to increase risks of anemia. Hospital Acquired Anemia (HAA), occurs when a patient admitted has no history of anemia but has anemia at discharge from the hospital. This may occur due to increased amount of blood drawn from the patient for phlebotomy purposes leading to anemia.

- **How it may be avoided:**
   a. Avoid drawing additional tubes.
   b. Check for the policy set by the facility for the amount of blood to be drawn according to patient's age and condition.

PARALYSIS (PARTIAL VS COMPLETE)

While performing phlebotomy, if a needle hits a nerve, it may cause partial or complete damage to the nerve. The symptoms would be sharp, tingling pain. Some causes of a nerve injury during phlebotomy may include, incorrect needle angle, incorrect amount of pressure applied while performing venipuncture (phlebotomy), incorrect location of puncture and etc. Phlebotomy technicians must always focus on the procedure they will be performing since a nerve damage may result in permanent damage (partial or completed paralysis) to the patient.

a. **What to do next:**
   - Do not advance the needle being used for the procedure any deeper, immediately remove the needle if the patient complains of such symptoms. Record and report to the facility supervisor or other personnel in charge and seek immediate help.

b. **How it may be avoided:**
   - Do not insert needle inappropriately into the patient's arm without confirming an underlying vein.

IMMUNE SYSTEM: INFECTION

The following may be a reason for infection resulting from the procedure:

a. Needle hitting a bone may cause infection.
b. Contaminated needle used for the procedure may cause infection.
c. Not cleaning the site as per the recommended standard protocol may cause infection.
d. Reusing the same supplies when moving from one patient to another.

   a. **How it may be avoided:**
      - Performing proper hand hygiene.
      - Using new needles.
      - Avoid using a needle if the packaging is not intact.
      - Proper standard protocol on cleaning the site and letting it air dry.
      - Using appropriate antiseptic solution recommended for the procedure.
      - Appropriately bandaging the puncture site.
      - The supplies and equipment used for phlebotomy should be free of any contaminants.
      - Avoid re-using supplies when moving from one patient to another.

SPECIMEN MAY BE REJECTED DUE TO:

1. Missing patient information.
2. No label on the specimen or label with missing information.
3. Specimen not properly processed (centrifuged).
4. Label information not matching with a requisition form.

5. Damaged tube and leaking specimen.

6. Specimen hemolyzed.

7. Clotted blood (in an anticoagulant tube).

8. Specimen contaminated depending on various factors.

9. Time sensitive specimen not processed in time.

10. Temperature sensitive specimen not handled as required.

11. Light sensitive specimen not protected from light.

12. Wrong tube used for blood collection.

13. Expired tube.

14. Insufficient quantity of blood collection.

15. Improper order of draw.

16. Missing specimen during transportation.

GENERAL PROCEDURAL STEPS: CORRECT VS INCORRECT

PATIENT IDENTIFICATION
CORRECT
Patient must be identified using the proper forms of identification. Minimum 2 identifiers are required. The acceptable identifier may include Patient Name, Date of Birth (DOB), and Patient ID number. Ask the patient to state their name and date of birth, compare the ID number with the ID number on the requisition form or label as applicable. Your facility may have a procedure that must be followed for patient identification prior to the blood collection procedure, follow your facility protocols.

INCORRECT
Phlebotomy Technician stating patient's name and date of birth followed by asking the patient to verify if the information stated by phlebotomy technician is correct or incorrect.

NOTE
Failure to properly identify the patient causes wrong diagnosis, mismanagement, wrong medication, & inappropriate treatment.

TOURNIQUET APPLICATION
CORRECT
- Tourniquet application is 3 to 4 inches proximal from the site selected (antecubital).

- Tourniquet disposed of after collection to avoid cross-contamination from patient to patient.
- Releasing tourniquet within 60 seconds or 1 minute.
- Using a latex free tourniquet.
- Using an appropriate size tourniquet.

INCORRECT
- Tourniquet application is 1 to 2 inches proximal from the site selected.
- Tourniquet application is too tight.
- Tourniquet application is too loose.
- Incorrect tourniquet application.
- Using latex tourniquet on patient allergic to latex.
- Improper knot while tying the tourniquet, making it difficult to untie.
- Tourniquet application for more than 60 second or 1 minute.
- Using a small size tourniquet on a large arm.

NOTE
Failure to untie tourniquet for more than 60 seconds may lead to hemolysis and incorrect test results.

VEIN SELECTION
CORRECT
- Select the most appropriate site for blood collection procedure.

INCORRECT
- Collecting blood specimen from above the IV site.
- Collecting blood specimen from a hematoma site.

NOTE
- The phlebotomy technician must be careful when selecting the site of blood collection.
- Puncturing an incorrect site may cause injury.
- Collecting blood from hematoma and IV site (above) may lead to incorrect test results.

DILATING THE VEIN
CORRECT
- Instruct the patient on making a light fist to dilate the vein.

INCORRECT
- Instruct the patient on clenching and unclenching the fist to dilate the vein.

NOTE
Clenching and unclenching the fist may lead to elevated levels of potassium (hyperkalemia).

SITE CLEANSING
CORRECT
- Clean the site using 70% isopropyl alcohol and allow it to air dry.
- If alcohol is not the recommended antiseptic, use povidone iodine.

INCORRECT
- Cleaning the site using 70% isopropyl alcohol and performing the procedure without letting the alcohol air-dry.
- Not using the proper antiseptic recommended for the procedure.

NOTE
Let the alcohol air dry to avoid inaccurate results.

NEEDLE SELECTION
CORRECT
- Perform the procedure using the proper gauge needle.

INCORRECT
- Perform the procedure using any gauge needle.

NOTE
Not using the proper needle size may lead to the specimen undergoing hemolysis or clotting.

ORDER OF DRAW
CORRECT
- Follow the correct order of draw for blood collection.

INCORRECT
- Collect the blood in any order of draw.

NOTE
Not following the correct order of draw may lead to mixing of additives and contamination of specimens. This may also lead to inaccurate results.

COLLECTION TUBES
CORRECT
- Use the proper size tube prefilled with vacuum, taking into consideration the size of the vein.

INCORRECT
- Use any size tube prefilled with vacuum, without taking into consideration the size of the vein.
- Using expired tubes.
- Not filling tube appropriately resulting in a short draw (additive to sample ratio are not proportional).
- Incorrect tube used for blood collection.
- Not storing the tube appropriately after blood collection.
- Vigorously shaking the tube after blood collection.

- Improper mixing of additive and collected blood.
- Not following the proper storage guidelines post blood collection.

NOTE
Not using the proper tube size prefilled with vacuum may cause the vein to collapse due to vacuum present in the tube.

SYRINGE COLLECTION
CORRECT
- While collecting the blood specimen, the plunger of the syringe must be pulled back gently.

INCORRECT
- While collecting the blood specimen, the plunger of the syringe must be pulled back abruptly.

NOTE
Abruptly pulling back of the plunger may cause hemolysis and may also cause the vein to collapse.

SPECIMEN DELIVERY
CORRECT
- Label the specimen appropriately.
- Double check the label applied to the specimen.
- Specimen collected is transported to the lab in an appropriate container or packaging within a timely manner.

INCORRECT
- Not labeling the specimen appropriately.
- Not transporting the specimen in a timely manner.
- Not packaging the specimen as per the recommended protocol.

NOTE
Not following the recommended protocols for specimen delivery may cause the specimen to be rejected by the lab and a redraw may be requested. If the test is performed on that specimen, it may provide inaccurate results.

TEST REQUISITION

A requisition is a form of document that contains information pertaining to the patient, specimen, provider, etc. It is also known as a request form. A requisition form gives the phlebotomy technician or the professional drawing the blood the information on the type of specimen to be drawn, the type of test to be performed and other pertinent information. The requisition form accompanies the specimen. The requisition form can either be electronically generated or manually prepared on a template that is available. It is recommended that you follow your facility guidelines. **The information that can be most commonly found on a requisition form would be:**

✓ Adequate patient identification information (e.g., full name, address, telephone number, medical record number)

✓ Unique Identification Number

✓ Patient gender

✓ Patient date of birth, or age

✓ Name and address of physician ordering the test

✓ Test(s) requested

✓ Date of specimen collection, when appropriate

✓ Source and type of specimen collected

✓ Time of collection

✓ Assay(s) performed

✓ Clinical & laboratory information, when appropriate

✓ Providers name

✓ Address of location (specimen collected)

✓ Billing information & other information as required.

PHLEBOTOMY ESSENTIALS:
OTHER PROCEDURES

In this section, we will discuss the following topics;

• Blood Collection from Pediatric and Neonates

• Blood Sugar Tests

• Blood Cultures

• Blood Collection for Legal Purposes

• Therapeutic Drug Monitoring (TDM)

• Urine Specimen Collection

• Stool Specimen Collection

• Sputum Specimen Collection

• Throat Swab Specimen Collection

• Blood Donation Procedure

BLOOD COLLECTION: PEDIATRIC AND NEONATES

Identification process: identify the patient correctly by either checking the patient's wrist or foot band. Verify the Patient's Name, Date of Birth, and ID Number on the requisition. Drawing blood from a pediatric patient requires proper skills and understanding of the procedure.

Blood drawn from a pediatric population must be done carefully since the Pediatric patient has less amount of blood than an elderly patient. The patient's age must be taken into consideration in reference to the quantity of blood to be collected to avoid anemia or some serious effects of excessive blood withdrawal.

The behavior of pediatric population may vary from patient to patient: some pediatric patients may have a fear of needle, while others may not. There are several types of behavior that pediatric patient displays such as fear of either strangers or pain, or maybe both, or may be due to their past experience. When approaching, be friendly with the patient and talk to them in a calm manner, show respect and be polite in the way you approach them.

Preparing the patient: Have another phlebotomist or parent assist you while performing the procedure. The patient's arm must be stationary, and not moving to draw a blood sample. Follow your facility policy on correct arm position of the pediatric patient.

Blood collection from pediatric population may cause the following:

• Anemia

• Damage to surrounding tissue.

• Infection

• Bleeding

PEDIATRIC BLOOD COLLECTION PROCEDURE BY AGE

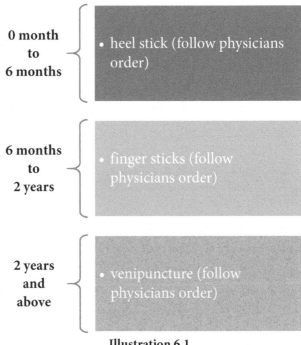

Illustration 6.1

Follow your facility policy on using the proper technique most appropriate to the patient's age.

BLOOD COLLECTION QUANTITY FROM PEDIATRIC POPULATION:

Drawing an excess amount of blood from a pediatric patient can cause serious complications. Facilities usually determine the level of blood that should be collected on the basis of the patient's age and weight. Collecting blood more than the normal quantity determined, may cause harmful effects. The phlebotomy technician must ensure to review the volume of blood that must be drawn from the pediatric patient prior to performing the blood draw.

Note: Follow your facility policy and guidelines on drawing blood from the pediatric population.

GENERAL PRECAUTIONS FOR PEDIATRIC DERMAL PUNCTURE

- Avoid a deep puncture.
- Avoid areas that are injured or swollen.
- Do not keep harmful equipment and supply in close vicinity to the patient.
- Avoid reusing the lancet.

NEONATAL SCREENING COLLECTION

In the United States of America, all newborns are screened. Newborn screening is a procedure that is performed on a newborn to identify conditions that the newborn might have. If identified, may assist the provider(s) in performing the treatment. Early detection of the condition by performing newborn screening helps in the future development of the newborn. The tests of the neonates differ from state to state. The newborn screening test has the capability to screen for 50 plus conditions. The test is performed within 48 hours of birth and also after that as per the recommendation. The most basic screening includes screening for congenital hypothyroidism, galactosemia, and phenylketonuria (PKU). The procedure involves collecting the blood on a special newborn screen card and sending it to the lab for further analysis.

PROCEDURE FOR NEONATAL SCREENING USING A FILTER PAPER

1. Gather all equipment and supplies.
2. Identify the patient.
3. Follow the standard protocols as per the recommended guidelines (follow your facility policy)
   - Perform a heel puncture.
   - The first drop of the blood from the heel puncture must be wiped away.
   - Next, fill the circle of the filter paper by touching a sufficient drop of blood to fill the circle completely. Do not touch area within the circle. Only the drop of blood should come in direct contact with the filter paper.
   - Keep the filter paper away from sunlight.
   - Let it dry for recommended time frame. The filter paper must be placed horizontally when drying the filter paper.

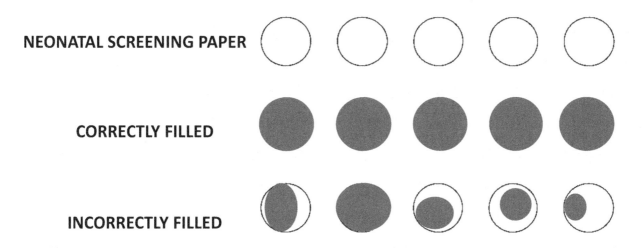

Figure 6.5 NEONATAL SCREENING

BLOOD SUGAR TESTS

FASTING BLOOD SUGAR

- If a fasting specimen is required, ask the patient about the last time they ingested food or liquid.
- The patient should be instructed to avoid eating for 8 hours or more, as recommended by the provider.
- Follow your facility policy on recommended hours the patient must not eat or drink any liquid, except water.

RANDOM BLOOD SUGAR

In this type of blood test, the blood is collected during any time of the day to check the sugar level of the blood.

2-HOUR POSTPRANDIAL (PP) TEST

This test determines the level of blood sugar in a person by comparing the fasting blood sugar to 2 hours postprandial (post-meal) blood sugar. **Prandial** means related to meal. **Post** means after.

- **In a regular person, the blood sugar level may be normal.**
- **In a person with diabetes, the blood sugar level may be elevated.**

ORAL GLUCOSE TOLERANCE TEST (OGTT)

A predetermined amount of glucose is provided to the person that must be ingested by mouth.

Types of GTT are
– 2 Hour Glucose Tolerance Test
– 3 Hour Glucose Tolerance Test
– 5 Hour Glucose Tolerance Test

Follow the physician's order on the type of test to be performed. A fasting specimen may be requested first before performing the Glucose Tolerance Test.

For 2 Hour Glucose Tolerance Test
- First specimen collected 1 hour after ingesting glucose.
- Second specimen collected 2 hours after ingesting glucose.

For 3 Hour Glucose Tolerance Test
- First specimen collected 1 hour after ingesting glucose.
- Second specimen collected 2 hours after ingesting glucose.
- Third specimen is collected 3 hours after ingesting glucose.

For 5 Hour Glucose Tolerance Test
- First specimen collected 1 hour after ingesting glucose.
- Second specimen collected 2 hours after ingesting glucose.
- Third specimen is collected 3 hours after ingesting glucose.
- Fourth specimen is collected 4 hours after ingesting glucose.
- Fifth specimen is collected 5 hours after ingesting glucose.

Figure 6.5

BLOOD CULTURES (BC)

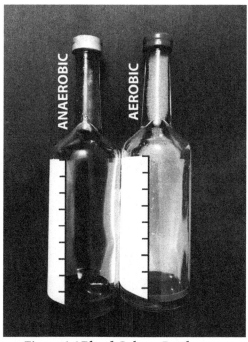

Figure 6.6 Blood Culture Bottles

Blood culture are tests that are performed to detect the presence of bacteria, or fungi in the blood. It is usually ordered when the provider suspects the presence of infection in the blood. The procedure involves drawing blood in blood culture containers (bottles) and sending it to the laboratory for further analysis.

Two samples are collected in separate bottles

✓ First Collected Sample Bottle 1 (Anaerobic: Absence of Air)
✓ Second Collected Sample Bottle 2 (Aerobic: Presence of Air)

Special precautions must be practiced to avoid contamination of the collected sample.

PROCEDURE TO PERFORM BLOOD CULTURE

COMPETENCY CHECKLIST: COLLECTING BLOOD FOR BLOOD CULTURE

PREPARATION PHASE

1. Verifying Physician's Order.
- Depending on the facility, the phlebotomy technician might be required to read the requisition form first before proceeding to perform the procedure.
- The requisition form provides the phlebotomy technician the information about the type of procedure that is to be performed, the patient's information and other information relevant to the procedure. Therefore, read the requisition form correctly.

2. Greeting, identifying yourself, & identifying the patient (full name & date of birth).
- Greeting your patient should be done as part of work ethics. Greet and identify yourself to the patient.
- Identify patient by asking the patient's name and date of birth. More identifiers may be required according to the policy of the facility.
- Identifying the patient is a crucial step of the procedure, as improper identification may lead to potential medical errors.

3. Assembling equipment and supplies.
- Gather all the equipment and supplies required for performing the procedure.
- Mark the bottle with the desired level of the specimen to be collected in the bottle as requested.
- Wipe the bottle top with isopropyl alcohol prep pads and allow it to dry.

4. Washing hands/donning PPE.
- Washing hands are performed as part of standard precautions.
- Select appropriate size gloves and don gloves.

5. Explaining procedure to the patient.
- Explaining the procedure prepares the patient for the procedure.
- The patient has the right to know about the procedure that they will be going through. Finally receive the consent from the patient for the procedure.
- Let the patient know that he/she will feel a small sting or pinch-like sensation when the needle is inserted into the site.

6. Positioning patient comfortably.
- Make sure that the patient is in a comfortable position.

7. Checking to review if the patient is on medication restrictions.
- Check for any medication (aspirin, warfarin or heparin or others); as some medications may increase the bleeding time.
- Follow your facility policy if the patient is on medication before the procedure is performed.

PROCEDURE PHASE
TOURNIQUET APPLICATION

8. Applying tourniquet at the appropriate location.

- Should be applied correctly 3 to 4 inches proximal to the incision site.
- It should not be excessively/extremely tight or excessively/extremely loose, nor should it cause discomfort to the patient.
  a) Application if excessively/extremely tight may decrease the flow of blood to the region and also result in petechiae.
  b) Application if excessively/extremely loose may not generate enough pressure for the vein to become prominent.

SITE SELECTION

9. Selecting incision site & palpate.

- Incision site should be carefully selected.

10. Removing tourniquet.

- Remove the tourniquet after the site has been selected. The phlebotomy technician may also directly proceed to the next step without removing the tourniquet. It is recommended that this step is performed during training sessions or until the technique is appropriately performed. **Note: Follow the facility guidelines.**

11. Scrubbing site using povidone iodine or chlorhexidine gluconate.

- Scrub site using Povidone iodine or chlorhexidine gluconate. The applicator must be scrubbed onto the puncture site for the recommended duration.

12. Connecting butterfly needle to the blood culture adapter, inspect needle (use appropriate gauge needle).

- Select an appropriate gauge needle for the procedure.
- Check to see if the needle has a manufacturing defect such as
  a) Damaged needle point, needle bevel or needle shaft.

13. Reapplying tourniquet.

- Should be applied correctly 3 to 4 inches proximal to the incision site.

NEEDLE INSERTION/SITE PUNCTURE

14. With the fingers (thumb or forefinger) of the non-butterfly needle unit carrying hand, pulling the skin taut below the site of the puncture.

15. With the butterfly needle unit carrying hand, inserting the needle at an appropriate angle.

- An appropriate angle must be chosen (15 degrees to 30 degrees angle)
- The bevel of the needle must face up when the needle is inserted.

16. Connecting the blood culture adapter to the blood culture bottle and allowing it to fill.

- Collect the sample in the anaerobic bottle first, followed by aerobic bottle second.

17. Removing the aerobic bottle before removing the needle.

18. Removing the needle and turning on (initiating) the safety device.

19. Applying direct pressure on incision site with a 2x2 gauze pad.

20. Disposing of sharps into a sharps container.

TUBE HANDLING AND LABELING

21. Performing blood culture bottle inversions by following the facility policy.

22. Labeling of the Blood culture bottles must be performed as per the facility policy.

- Check facility policy on labeling blood culture bottles.

PATIENT CARE

23. Checking on the patient for hemostasis by inspecting the site of the puncture.

24. Applying bandage once the bleeding stops.

SPECIMEN TRANSPORTATION

25. Packaging specimen for transport.

- Follow proper specimen packaging and transporting standards.

GLOVE REMOVAL, DISPOSAL AND HAND HYGIENE

26. Removing gloves using the proper technique of glove removal.

27. Disposing of gloves and other supplies into their appropriate containers.

28. Washing hands using the proper technique of hand washing.

DOCUMENTATION

29. Documenting the procedure electronically or manually.

- Follow your facility policy on documenting the procedure.

BLOOD COLLECTION FOR LEGAL PURPOSES

a. Use an appropriate blood collection kit, if available.

b. Explain procedure and obtain consent prior to performing the blood collection.

c. The blood sample collected must be sealed appropriately according to the recommended guidelines.

d. Do not use alcohol for cleaning the site, if the test is being performed to check blood alcohol levels.

The blood sample container label may include the following information as required:

1. Complete name of the subject.

2. Name of the facility submitting the sample.

3. Address where the blood sample was drawn.

4. Name of the phlebotomy technician collecting the blood sample.

5. Date and time at which the blood was collected.

6. Witnessing officer initials or signature present at the time of collection according to the recommended guidelines.

7. A Chain of possession on a form that shows the persons involved in handling the evidence.

Note: additional information may be required. Follow your facility policy on labeling samples for legal purposes.

Chain of custody contains the complete paper trail of the evidence. It should identify: who, what, why, when, where, and how of specimen handling from start to the end of the procedure. Every move of the evidence should be in the chain of custody.

Some information that should be in the chain of custody should be as follows:

✓ A description of the evidence.

✓ List of any procedure or test done.

✓ From whom it was collected.

✓ Name and signature of the responsible person who handled the evidence.

✓ Every move of the evidence with the signature of each person involved in handling the evidence.

✓ Date and time it was collected, stored or transferred.

✓ Where was it stored and by whom, when, and why?

THERAPEUTIC DRUG MONITORING (TDM)

1. **Therapeutic** means for treatment purposes.
2. **Drug** refers to the prescription drug
3. **Monitoring** means to observe, track, keep under observation, etc.

A physician orders a therapeutic drug monitoring (TDM) for the patient. Therapeutic drug monitoring is performed to monitor the concentrations of the drug in the blood.

Therapeutic drug monitoring (TDM) monitors to check if the level of prescribed drug is

Under or above the therapeutic ranges

1. Under the therapeutic range may be ineffective due to under-dosing.
2. Above the therapeutic range may be toxic due to overdosing.

Overview of the Therapeutic Drug Monitoring (TDM) process:

1. The physician requests the therapeutic drug monitoring (TDM).
2. The blood sample is drawn at a timed interval.
3. Laboratory measures the levels of the drug found from the collected timed blood sample.
4. Levels of the drug measured are reported to the physician.
5. The physician interprets the results.

URINALYSIS

The urinalysis is used as a screening and/or diagnostic tool to detect abnormal findings in the urine sample.

Three components of the test:

1. Physical Examination
2. Chemical Examination
3. Microscopic Examination

PHYSICAL EXAMINATION

URINE: Appearance
URINE: Volume
URINE: Odor

Illustration 6.3

APPEARANCE: COLOR

Normal color:

PALE YELLOW OR

COLORLESS URINE

URINE: APPEARANCE

Clarity: Normal urine can be clear or cloudy

Abnormal Clarity:

1. Clear Urine
2. Slightly Cloudy Urine
3. Cloudy Urine

URINE VOLUME

The average adult: 1000ml to 2000ml/24hours

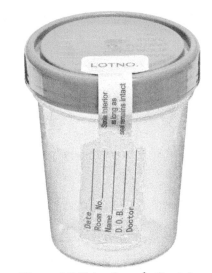

Figure 6.7 Urine Sample Container

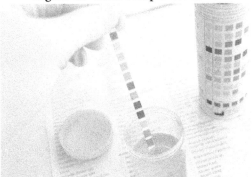

Figure 6.8 DipStick dipped into urine specimen

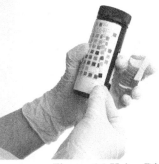

Figure 6.9 Urine DipStick

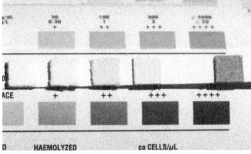

Figure 6.9a

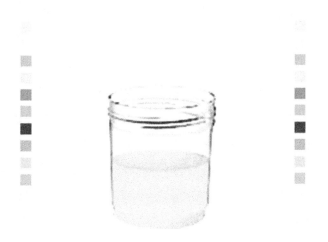

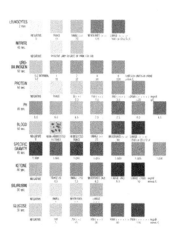

Test Strip Before Dipping	Urine Sample	Test Strip After Dipping	Compare the Test Strip After Dipping with the Above Chart

CHEMICAL EXAMINATION

1. Urine PH
2. Protein
3. Glucose
4. Ketones
5. Occult blood
6. Bilirubin
7. Urobilinogen
8. Nitrites
9. Leukocytes
10. Specific Gravity

URINE PH

Normal PH: The average is approximately 6
Higher PH: Alkaline Urine
Lower PH: Acid Urine

PROTEIN IN URINE

Normal: About or below 150 mg/24 hours.
Abnormal: Above 150 mg/day.

GLUCOSE IN URINE

Normal: Absent
Abnormal: Present

KETONES IN URINE

Normal: Absent
Abnormal: Present

BLOOD IN URINE

Normal: Absent
Abnormal: Present

BILIRUBIN IN URINE

Normal: Absent
Abnormal: Present

UROBILINOGEN IN URINE

Normal: Present (in low concentration)
Abnormal: Present (in high concentration)

NITRITES IN URINE

Normal: Absent
Abnormal: Present

LEUKOCYTES

Normal: Very Few
Abnormal: Significant presence of infection (White Blood Cells)

SPECIFIC GRAVITY (SG)

Reflects the density of the urine.
Range of 1.001 to 1.040

Increase in SG:
urine volume↓ and SG↑

Decrease in SG:
urine volume↑ and SG ↓

URINE SPECIMEN COLLECTION

Urine Specimen Types

Mid-Stream Clean Catch:

The patient should be educated about cleansing the urethral area.

MALE: Clean the penis in a circumcised penis. If uncircumcised, then instruct the patient to retract the skin and clean the penis (proximal). While holding the retracted skin, void the first part (stream) of the urine into the toilet and then place the cup to collect the urine (mid-stream clean catch). On completion, place the lid on the container to seal the container.

FEMALE: Hold the labia's apart and clean the labia on one side, from front to back, then on the other side of the labia from front to back. Finally, clean the center of the labia. While holding the labia apart, void the first portion of the urine into the toilet and then place the cup to collect the urine (mid-stream clean catch). On completion, place the lid on the container to seal the container.
Specimens after collection should be labeled correctly with the required information, and transported to the lab for analysis.

Timed Specimen (24 Hour Collection):

The patient is provided with a container to collect the urine for the next 24 hours and instructions are provided on when to start the 24 hour collection time and when to stop. Instruct the patient to avoid fecal contamination of the urine sample.

Procedure for collection:

The patient is asked to urinate the first-morning urine into the toilet and start the 24 hr. urine test. After urination, record the time and date. Continue collecting urine in the urine container for the next 24 hours.

First Morning Sample/First Voided Specimen:

This specimen is considered to be a specimen of choice for examination, due to the sample being concentrated in form. The sample is free of any dietary influences. The patient is instructed to empty the bladder (pass urine) before bedtime and collect the first-morning sample (urine). This is a preferred collection for various types of analysis.

Random:

Most commonly used sample for urinalysis examination. The specimen can be collected at any time during the day from the patient. Random urine specimen can give inaccurate results depending on the patient's health. The patient is instructed to avoid contamination of the sample.

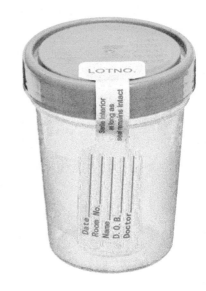

Figure: Urine Sample Container

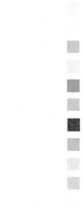

Figure: Urine Dip-Stick

AECA: Physical & Chemical Urinalysis Competency Check

Steps	Performed	Not Performed
1. Gather the required equipment and supplies.		
2. Review and verify physician's order.		
3. Perform hand hygiene and don PPE (follow standard precautions).		
4. Greet the patient.		
5. Identify yourself (name & designation).		
6. Identify patient (full name & date of birth).		
7. Explain procedure to the patient.		
8. Instruct patient in specimen collection.		
9. Perform physical urinalysis.		
10. Perform chemical urinalysis.		
11. Dispose of contaminated supplies into their respective containers.		
12. Perform hand hygiene.		
13. Document results into the patient's chart according to the facility policy.		

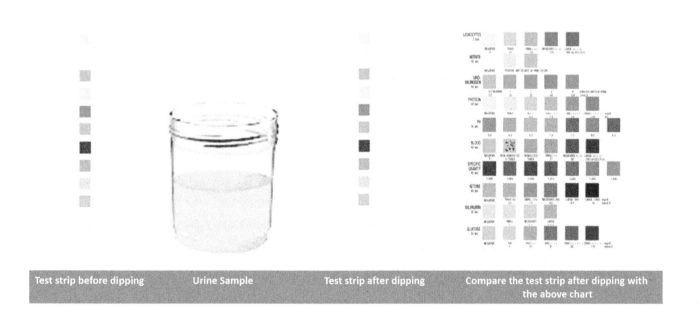

| Test strip before dipping | Urine Sample | Test strip after dipping | Compare the test strip after dipping with the above chart |

Stool Specimen Collection

FECAL SPECIMEN COLLECTION

3 TYPES OF FECAL TEST:

1. **Fecal occult blood test (FOBT)**

2. **Fecal immunochemical test (FIT), also called an immunochemical fecal occult blood test (iFOBT)**

3. **Stool DNA test (sDNA)**

Specimen collection methods:

✓ **Method 1:** Collection in a container.
✓ **Method 2:** Collection on a hemoccult card.

COLLECTION IN A CONTAINER:

- Gather your equipment and supplies.
- Don PPE (gloves)
- Uncap the collection container.
- Using a clean tongue blade, transfer the stool specimen from a bed pan or any other container in which it is initially present to the specimen collection container.
- Once the transfer is performed.
- Discard the tongue blade into a disposable bag.
- Next, cap the specimen collection container.
- Check for color and abnormality of the stool sample if any. Check the

HEMOCCULT COLLECTION CARD

Patient Name: _____ Patient Name: _____ Patient Name: _____
Age:_____ Age:_____ Age:_____
Address:_____ Address:_____ Address:_____
Sample Collected Date:_____ Sample Collected Date:_____ Sample Collected Date:_____
Phone Number:_____ Phone Number:_____ Phone Number:_____
Physician Name:_____ Physician Name:_____ Physician Name:_____

A   B   A   B   A   B

1   2   3

patient's information on the specimen container.

- Next, place the stool specimen collected into a biohazard bag.
- Finally, discard all disposable supplies into their appropriate container.
- Wash hands and record the procedure as per the facility protocols.

Note: The fecal specimen must be obtained according to the instructions provided. The container used to collect the fecal specimen must be clean.

COLLECTION ON A HEMO-CCULT CARD:

The stool specimen collected is to be applied to the designated areas of the fecal specimen collection card. This

is done by collecting the specimen and using the fecal collection card kit. Using the applicator, that is a part of the kit, immerse the applicator into the stool collected, and apply a layer of the stool onto the area designated; **Area A and Area B of Card 1**. Next, if more specimens are required, do the same for the second specimen. However, for this specimen, use **Area A and Area B of Card 2**. If the 3rd specimen is requested, perform the same step again, and collect the specimen onto Area A and Area B of Card 3. On collection of the specimen onto the card, close the card and dispose all the disposable supplies into their appropriate container.

SPUTUM COLLECTION
PROCEDURAL STEPS

1. Start by identifying the patient.

2. Gather all your equipment and supplies required to perform the procedure.

3. Explain the procedure to the patient.

4. Position the patient comfortably.

5. Ask the patient to rinse the mouth with water.

   i) Instruct the patient to breath in and out three times.

   ii) Instruct the patient to cough and bring the mucous from the lungs up into the oral cavity.

6. Open the container and transfer the sputum from the mouth into the container.

7. Close the lid of the container, label specimen appropriately and refrigerate until ready for transport to the lab.

8. Discard all the disposable supplies into their appropriate waste containers.

9. Thank the patient.

10. Document the procedure.

THROAT SWAB COLLECTION
EQUIPMENT & SUPPLIES
- ✓ A tongue depressor.
- ✓ Personal protective equipment.
- ✓ A sterile swab sticks with cotton tip applicator.
- ✓ A transport tube.

PROCEDURAL STEPS

1. Start by identifying the patient

2. Gather all your equipment and supplies required to perform the procedure.

3. Explain the procedure to the patient.

4. Position the patient comfortably.

5. Ask the patient to open his/her mouth.

6. Use a tongue depressor to depress the tongue.

7. Next, advance the sterile swab stick with cotton tip applicator into the patient's oral cavity.

8. Swab the lateral walls of the pharynx in the tonsillar area. This must be performed carefully without touching the tongue or other parts of the oral cavity.

9. Instruct the patient to open the mouth widely.

10. Withdraw the swab stick.

11. Place the swab stick into a transport tube or appropriate container as recommended.

12. Label specimen appropriately.

13. Discard all the disposable supplies into their appropriate waste containers.

14. Thank the patient.

15. Document the procedure.

Note: Follow your facility recommended protocol and policy on sputum and throat swab collection.

BLOOD DONATION

PRESCREENING

The individual should be screened before donating blood.

Donor Age: specified by the state.

Donor Weight: For whole blood collection, the minimum weight of the donor should be 110 lb.

Donor Health Status: Healthy (should not be on alcohol or drugs).

Donor Hemoglobin Level: Must be normal.

Donor Body Temperature: Normal body temperature.

Donor Blood Pressure: Should be within normal ranges.

Donor Pulse: Should be 50 – 100 beats per minute.

Note: It is crucial to check your facility guidelines and policy on;

- **Prescreening individuals for blood donation and**
- **Properly performing the procedure.**

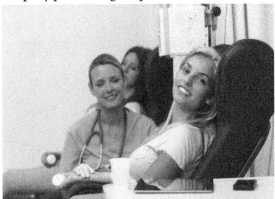

Figure 6.10

Donor Deferral means an individual disqualified for donating blood. Deferral can be permanent or temporary, depending on the reason for disqualification. If the individual is deferred temporarily, then he or she may not be able to donate the blood until the end of the deferred period.

Types of blood donation

Autologous and Directed Donation

AUTOLOGOUS: In this type of blood donation, the blood may be donated by the donor for his or her use.

DIRECTED DONATION: In this type of blood donation, the blood may be donated by an individual (family, friend, etc.) other than the donor for his or her use.

COLLECTING BLOOD FOR BLOOD DONATION

Follow the venipuncture procedure as recommended and use the below steps as per requirements

Step 1.   Assemble Equipment & Supplies

Step 2.   Perform hand hygiene

Step 3.   Identify donor and label blood collection bag and test tubes

Step 4.   Select the vein

Step 5.   Apply Blood Pressure Cuff at 40-60 mm Hg

Step 6.   Disinfect the skin

- If using 2% chlorhexidine gluconate in 70% isopropyl alcohol, the solution should be in contact for 30 seconds.

- If 2% chlorhexidine gluconate in 70% isopropyl alcohol is not available, apply 70% isopropyl alcohol and allow it to dry for 30 seconds which is followed by use of tincture iodine or chlorhexidine 2% and allow it to dry for 30 seconds.

Step 7.   Perform the venipuncture: use 16-18 gauge needle as recommended by the facility. The donor should be asked to open and close the fist as recommended by the facility.

Step 8.   Monitor the donor and the collected blood

Step 9.   Remove the needle & perform care for puncture site by applying firm pressure over the puncture site using gauze.

Step 10. After a blood donation: The donor should be allowed to rest for some time, meanwhile, check for signs of bleeding and fainting. Some donors may show postural hypotension due to the removal of blood leading to a low blood pressure. Donating blood usually only takes 45-60 minutes.

Safety Data Sheet (SDS)

Safety Data Sheets (SDS) was formerly known as Material Safety Data Sheets or MSDSs. **SAFETY DATA SHEET** is required to be provided by the manufacturer or related entities for each hazardous chemical so that the user have information on the product they may be using. Safety data sheet is a set of information that provides information on identification, ingredients, physical and chemical properties. It further provides information on first aid measures that can be taken and fire fighting measures that can be taken. Apart from these, it also has information on handling and storage, accidental release and exposure protection. Other information includes stability, reactivity, and toxicological information. Additional information may also be available on the safety data sheet.

Reference: https://www.osha.gov/Publications/OSHA3514.html

INCIDENT REPORT

An incident is an unusual occurrence of an accident. An incident can occur during patient care. If it occurs, it must be documented properly accordingly to the recommended guidelines. The purpose of the incident report is to document the details of the event or occurrence of an accident as soon as possible. For example; a patient falls while walking within the hospital, this accident may be reported on the incident report. Check your healthcare facility policy on documenting incident report. General information that may be required to fill the incident report may include but not limited to the following:

- Location and Name of the facility.
- Name of the person involved in the accident.
- Time of incident including AM or PM.
- Type of accident.
- Witness name(s).
- Description summary of the incident.
- Action taken for patient care.
- Other information as required by the facility.

PROFESSIONAL LIABILITY INSURANCE

The facilities liability insurance may cover the phlebotomist. However, the phlebotomy technician may get themselves insured by a professional liability insurance also known as "**PLI**."

A phlebotomist must understand that the phlebotomy procedure is an invasive procedure and may involve risk if not performed properly. Each facility has their own policies and procedures to ensure that phlebotomy procedures are performed as safely and correctly as possible. The injuries to the patient may cause nerve damage, infection, hematoma, tendon injury, soft tissue injury, bone infection and more. A phlebotomist should be very careful while performing the procedure and not perform the procedure if he or she is not trained for it. Sometimes, even performing the procedure correctly may lead to an injury. A standard of care should always be followed when performing a phlebotomy procedure. Make sure that you follow the established standard of care.

FEW STEPS TO MINIMIZE ERRORS FOR PHLEBOTOMIST:

- Proper communication with the patient.
- Be attentive before, during and after the procedure.
- Obtaining an informed consent describing the risk involved in the procedure.
- Have proper training on skills that will be performed.
- Have the appropriate knowledge of the procedure.
- If you have a question regarding the procedure, ask the doctor, supervisor or the appropriate person in your facility.
- Follow appropriate and established standard of care.
- Maintain proper documentation.
- Proper patient identification.
- Proper site selection.
- Perform duties within the scope of practice.
- Provide appropriate information to the patient required for the procedure.
- Report incident to the supervisor and fill out an incident report.

- Follow your facility recommended guidelines on performing the procedure and other guidelines as applicable.

FEW CAUSES OF LIABILITY INVOLVING PHLEBOTOMIST

- Improper identification of the patient, leading to misdiagnosis and erroneous treatment causing injury and serious risk to patient's life.

- Failure to draw the blood sample appropriately.
- Breaching patient's privacy.
- Damage caused to the patient as a direct result of phlebotomy procedure.
- Not following sterile technique, leading to patient infection.
- Improper handling technique after the specimen is collected from the patient.
- Using an improper needle, leading to an injury.

CHAPTER 6

END OF CHAPTER REVIEW QUESTIONS

Question Set 1: Match the following

Column A	Answer	Column B
1. Excessive bleeding		A. small spot on the skin, red or purple in color, caused by hemorrhage to the capillary (blood vessel).
2. Uncooperative patient		B. this can occur as a result of hitting an artery while performing venipuncture. The blood collected in the blood collection tube as a result of an arterial puncture would be pulsating and bright red in color.
3. Septicemia		C. Internal swelling of the vein due to repeated injury causes the vein to block temporarily leading to a collapsed vein. Another reason could be the vacuum in the blood collection tube may cause the vein to collapse, this may occur due to the size of the vein or other factors.
4. Petechiae		D. After the procedure, there may be excessive bleeding; it may be as a result of an improper technique or due to the patient having a condition that inhibits the clotting process (hemophilia).
5. Arterial puncture		E. It might sometimes be difficult to draw blood from infants and children or patients that are mentally not stable.
6. Collapsed vein		F. Not following the precautions and proper procedural standards such as (using contaminated equipment and supplies may cause infection in the blood.
7. Bone infection		G. Injury to a blood vessel leads to clot formation.
8. Inability to Draw Blood		H. A blood clot formed within the vein further cause's inflammation, redness, and pain. The most common affected veins are the veins that are located closer to the surface of the skin.
9. Compartmental syndrome		I. Improper handling of the needle during the procedure may cause injury to the skin and the underlying structures resulting in pain.
10. Seizures		J. An allergic response may initiate as a result of an equipment or supply used during the procedure. The most common supply that may initiate an allergic response would be using a latex glove.
11. Hematoma		K. Inflammation of vein may occur due to injury to that vein due to venipuncture or due to blood clot formation.
12. Allergic Response		L. A patient may faint (before, during or after the procedure).
13. Phlebitis		M. While performing phlebotomy, if a needle hits the nerve, it may cause partial or complete damage to the nerve. The symptoms would be sharp, tingling pain.

14. Hemolysis		N. A patient may undergo seizures while the procedure is being performed.
15. Syncope		O. Occurs due to injury caused by the needle insertion leading to accumulation of blood external to the blood vessels and within the tissue causing internal bleeding of the tissue.
16. Nerve Involvement		P. A breakdown of red blood cells. Breakdown of RBCs causes the release of hemoglobin.
17. Thrombus		Q. Increase in concentration of red blood cells and other formed elements.
18. Thrombo-phlebitis		R. A patient may experience this as a result of a shock or pain; it can lead to fainting.
19. Pain		S. While performing phlebotomy, if a bone is hit with either a needle or a lancet, it may cause_____
20. Vasovagal reaction		T. A phlebotomist may not be able to draw blood from a patient on the 1st attempt.
21. Hemoconcentration		U. This can occur as a result of excessive bleeding post-phlebotomy procedure. _____ occurs when more than normal pressure develops in a particular space within the human body.

TYPES OF TEST REQUEST (Match the following)

Column A	Answer	Column B
Timed		Requires immediate test results.
Routine		Requires test results as soon as possible but not immediately.
STAT		Requires test results (not immediately or as soon as possible).
Asap		A blood draw is performed at a specific time, and test results are reported as routine. If required as a STAT order, the results are required immediately.

Question Set 2: Essay Questions

1. Discuss about venipuncture site selection problems.
2. Discuss prevention of hemolysis.
3. Explain in brief the problems associated with tourniquet applications.
4. List possible complications that can occur during blood collection procedure.
5. Explain in brief about the compartmental syndrome.
6. Explain therapeutic drug monitoring.
7. Explain the procedure involved in blood collection for legal purposes.
8. Explain collection methods of different urine specimen types.

a. Mid-Stream Clean Catch
b. Timed Specimen (24 Hour Collection)
c. First Morning Sample/First Voided Specimen
d. Random urine sample

9. List the reasons for specimen rejection.
10. Explain about blood collection specimens that are:
   a. Time Sensitive
   b. Light Sensitive
   c. Temperature Sensitive
11. Explain in brief about petechiae, hemolysis, and hemoconcentration.

Question Set 3: Sequence in Order

STOOL COLLECTION IN A CONTAINER: Write the correct number next to the step in column A.

Column A	Column B
Uncap the collection container.	
Discard the tongue blade into a disposable bag.	
Check for color and abnormality of the stool sample if any. Check the patient's information on the specimen container.	
Next, place the stool specimen collected into a biohazard bag.	
Finally, discard all disposable supplies into their appropriate container.	

Using a clean tongue blade, transfer the stool specimen from a bed pan or any other container in which it is initially present to the specimen collection container.

Gather your equipment and supplies.

Don PPE (gloves)

Wash hands and record the procedure as per the facility protocols.

Once the transfer is performed.

Next, cap the specimen collection container.

THROAT SWAB COLLECTION PROCEDURE. Write the correct number next to the step in column A.

Column A	Column B
	Next, advance the sterile swab stick with cotton tip applicator into the patient's oral cavity.
	Swab the lateral walls of the pharynx in the tonsillar area. This must be performed carefully without touching the tongue or other parts of the oral cavity.
	Use a tongue depressor to depress the tongue.
	Start by identifying the patient
	Gather all your equipment and supplies required to perform the procedure.
	Instruct the patient to open the mouth widely.
	Ask the patient to open his/her mouth.
	Explain the procedure to the patient.
	Position the patient comfortably.
	Discard all the disposable supplies into their appropriate waste containers.
	Thank the patient.
	Document the procedure.
	Withdraw the swab stick.
	Place the swab stick into a transport tube or appropriate container as recommended.
	Label specimen appropriately.

Question Set 4: True or False (T/F)

1. Thrombophlebitis are small spot on the skin, red or purple in color, caused by hemorrhage to the capillary (blood vessel).
True or False
2. Septicemia is an allergic response may initiate as a result of an equipment or supply used during the procedure.
True or False
3. A hematoma occurs due to injury caused by the needle insertion leading to accumulation of blood external to the blood vessels and within the tissue causing internal bleeding of the tissue.
True or False
4. Hemolysis is an increase in the concentration of red blood cells and other formed elements.
True or False
5. Hemoconcentration is a breakdown of red blood cells.
True or False

APPENDIX A: ABBREVIATIONS

Ab: Antibody

ABG: Arterial blood gasses

Abn: Abnormal

ABN: Advanced beneficiary notice

ABO: Blood type

ACE: angiotensin converting enzyme

ACH: acetylcholine

Afib: Atrial fibrillation

Ag: Antigen

AIDS: Acquired immune deficiency syndrome

Alb: Albumin

ALKP: alkaline phosphatase

ALT: Alanine aminotransferase

APTT: Activated Partial Thromboplastin Time

ARDS: Adult respiratory distress syndrome

AST: aspartate aminotransferase

BASO: Basophil

Bact: Bacteria

BC: Blood culture

Bili: Bilirubin

BMP: Basic metabolic panel

BMT: Bone marrow transplant

BT: Bleeding time

BUN: blood urea nitrogen

Ca: Calcium

Cath: Catheterize

CBC: Complete blood count

CBCD: Complete blood count with differential

Cc: Cubic centimeters

CHF: Congestive heart failure

Chol: Cholesterol

CMP: Comprehensive metabolic panel

COPD: Chronic obstructive pulmonary disease

CPK: Creative phosphokinase

Creat: Creatinine

CRF: Chronic renal failure

CSF: Cerebrospinal fluid

C&S: Culture and sensitivity

CV: cell volume

CVA: Cerebrovascular accident

DD: Directed donor

DIC: Disseminated intravascular coagulation

dL: deciliters

DM: Diabetes mellitus

DOB: Date of birth

DVT: Deep vein thrombosis

Dx: Diagnosis

EBV: Epstein - Barr virus

E coli: Escherichia coli

EDTA: Ethylenediaminetetraacetic acid

EOS: Eosinophil

ER: Emergency room

ERP: Emergency room panel

ESR: Erythrocyte Sedimentation Rate

FBS: Fasting blood sugar

Fe: Iron

FFP: Fresh frozen plasma

GERD: Gastroesophageal reflux disease

g: grams

Glu: Glucose

GTT: Glucose tolerance test

HCG: Human Chorionic Gonadotropin

Hct: hematocrit

HDL: High-Density Lipoprotein

Hgb: hemoglobin

H&H: Hemoglobin and hematocrit

HIV: Human Immunodeficiency virus

HTN: Hypertension

ICU: Intensive care unit

ID: Identification

IgG: immunoglobulin G

IgM: immunoglobulin M

INR: International normalized ratio

IV: Intravenous

K: Potassium

kg: kilograms

L&D: Labor and delivery

LDH: Lactic acid dehydrogenase

LDL: Low-Density Lipoprotein

LFT: Liver function test

Li: Lithium

lt: liters

Lytes: Electrolytes

LYMPH: Lymphocyte

MCHC: Mean Cell Hemoglobin Concentration

MCV: Mean Cell Volume

mcg or µg: micrograms

mcl or µL: microliters

MCH: Mean Cell Hemoglobin

mEq: milliequivalents

mg: milligrams

MI: Myocardial infarction

mIu: milli-international units

mL: milliliters

mm³: cubic milliliters

mm: millimeter

Mmol: millimoles

MPV: Mean Platelet Volume

MRSA: Methicillin-resistant staphylococcus aureus

MSDA: Material safety data sheet

Na: Sodium

NEUT: Neutrophil

NP: Nasopharyngeal

NSAID: Nonsteroidal anti-inflammatory drugs

O₂: oxygen

OGTT: Oral Glucose Tolerance Test

O&P: Ova and parasites

OSHA: Occupational safety and health administration

Path: pathology

PKU: phenylketonuria

PLT: Platelet

POCT: point of care testing

PPE: personal protective equipment

PT: prothrombin time

PTT: partial thromboplastin time

PT/INR: Prothrombin Time/International Normalized Ratio

QA: quality assurance

QC: quality control

QNS: quantity no sufficient

RBC: Red Blood Cell (erythrocytes)

RF: Rheumatoid Factor

SGOT: serum glutamic-oxaloacetic transaminase

SGPT: serum glutamic pyruvic transaminase

SST: serum separator tube

Stat: immediately

STAP: Staphylococcus

STREP: Streptococcus

TAT: turn around time

TIA: transient ischemic attack

TSH: Thyroid Stimulating Hormone

UA: urinalysis

µL: microliter

UTI: urinary tract infection

U: units

WBC: White Blood Cell (Leukocyte)

APPENDIX B: BLOOD TEST PANELS

Basic metabolic panel (Calcium, ionized)

Calcium, ionized
Carbon dioxide
Chloride
Creatinine
Glucose
Potassium
Sodium
Urea Nitrogen

Basic metabolic panel (Calcium, total)

Calcium, ionized
Carbon dioxide
Chloride
Creatinine
Glucose
Potassium
Sodium
Urea Nitrogen (BUN)

General health panel

Comprehensive metabolic panel
Blood count, complete (CBC), automated and appropriate manual differential WBC count
Thyroid stimulating hormone

Electrolyte panel

Carbon dioxide
Chloride
Potassium
Sodium

Comprehensive metabolic panel

Albumin
Bilirubin, total
Calcium, total
Carbon dioxide (bicarbonate)
Chloride
Creatinine
Glucose
Phosphatase, alkaline
Potassium
Protein, total
Sodium
Transferase, alanine amino (ALT) (SGPT)

Transferase, aspartate amino (AST)
Urea nitrogen (BUN)

Obstetric panel

Blood count, complete (CBC), automated and automated differential WBC count
Hepatitis B surface antigen (HBsAG)
Antibody, rubella
Syphilis test, non-treponemal antibody; qualitative (e.g., VDRL, RPR, ART)
Antibody screen, RBC, each serum technique
Blood typing, ABO
Blood typing, Rh (D)

Lipid panel

Cholesterol, serum, total
Lipoprotein, direct measurement, high-density cholesterol (HDL cholesterol)
Triglycerides

Renal function panel

Albumin
Calcium, total
Carbon dioxide (bicarbonate)
Chloride
Creatinine
Glucose
Phosphorus inorganic (phosphate)
Potassium
Sodium
Urea nitrogen (BUN)

Acute hepatitis panel

Hepatitis A antibody (HAAb), IgM antibody
Hepatitis B core antibody (HBcAB), IgM antibody
Hepatitis B surface antigen (HBsAg)
Hepatitis C antibody

Hepatic function panel

Albumin
Bilirubin, total
Bilirubin, direct
Phosphate, alkaline
Protein, total
Transferase, alanine amino (ALT) (SGPT)
Transferase, aspartate amino (AST) (SGOT)

APPENDIX C: BASIC ABBREVIATIONS AND CONVERSIONS

ABBREVIATIONS	
gal or gals	gallons
O, pt or pts	pints
oz or ozs	ounces
fl.oz	fluid ounces
lb or lbs	pounds
cl	centilitre ($1/_{100}$ L)
ml	milliliter ($1/_{1000}$ L)
µl	microlitre ($1/_{1,000,000}$ L)
meq or mEq	Milliequivalent
m	meter
mm	millimeter ($1/_{1,000}$ m)
cc or cu.cm	cubic centimeters ($1/_{1,000}$ L)
g	gram
kg	kilogram (1,000g)
mg	milligram ($1/_{1,000}$g)
mcg or µg	microgram ($1/_{1,000,000}$g)
L or l	liter

APPROXIMATE EQUIVALENCIES	
1 liter	**1000 milliliter**
1 liter	10 deciliter
1 deciliter	**100 milliliter**
1 milliliter	1000 microliter
1 milliliter	**1 cubic centimeters**
1 cubic centimeters	1 gram or 1 milliliter (approx.)
1 kilogram	**1000 grams**
1 kilogram	2.2 pounds
1 gram	**100mg**
454 grams	1 pound
1,000 milliliters	**1 ounce**
1,000 liters	1 kiloliter
1 gallon	**3.79 liters or 3790 milliliter**
1 pint	0.48 liters (or 480 milliliters)

APPENDIX D: SAMPLE BLOOD REPORT WITH NORMAL RANGES: RANGES MAY VARY

```
Tests: (1) CBC With Differential/Platelet (005009)        Normal Range
   WBC                                                     3.4-10.8
   RBC                                                     3.77-5.28
   Hemoglobin                                              11.1-15.9
   Hematocrit                                              34.0-46.6
   MCV                     [L]                             79-97
   MCH                     [L]                             26.6-33.0
   MCHC                                                    31.5-35.7
   RDW                                                     12.3-15.4
   Platelets                                               155-379
   Neutrophils                                             40-74
   Lymphs                  [H]                             14-46
   Monocytes                                               4-12
   Eos                                                     0-5
   Basos                                                   0-3
 ! Immature Cells
  Neutrophils (Absolute)
                                                           1.4-7.0
   Lymphs (Absolute)       [H]                             0.7-3.1
   Monocytes(Absolute)                                     0.1-0.9
   Eos (Absolute)                                          0.0-0.4
   Baso (Absolute)                                         0.0-0.2
 ! Immature Granulocytes
                                                           0-2
 ! Immature Grans (Abs)                                    0.0-0.1
 ! NRBC
   Hematology Comments:


Tests: (2) Comp. Metabolic Panel (14) (322000)
   Glucose, Serum                                          65-99
   BUN                                                     6-20
   Creatinine, Serum                                       0.57-1.00
 ! eGFR If NonAfricn Am                                    >59
 ! eGFR If Africn Am                                       >59
   BUN/Creatinine Ratio [H]                                8-20
   Sodium, Serum                                           134-144
   Potassium, Serum                                        3.5-5.2
   Chloride, Serum                                         97-108
  Carbon Dioxide, Total
                                                           19-28
   Calcium, Serum                                          8.7-10.2
  Protein, Total, Serum
                                                           6.0-8.5
   Albumin, Serum                                          3.5-5.5
   Globulin, Total                                         1.5-4.5
 ! A/G Ratio                                               1.1-2.5
   Bilirubin, Total                                        0.0-1.2
  Alkaline Phosphatase, S
                                                           39-117
   AST (SGOT)                                              0-40
   ALT (SGPT)                                              0-32
```

APPENDIX E: SAMPLE PHLEBOTOMY REQUISITION FORM

SAMPLE PHLEBOTOMY REQUISITION FORM

INFORMATION: PATIENT

| Last Name | | First Name | | SSN | | D.O.B. | | M ☐ |
| | | | | | | | | F ☐ |

| Street Address | | Apt# | City | | State | ZIP | | Phone |

INFORMATION: SPECIMEN

Date of order: ___ / ___ / ___

Requested start date: ___ / ___ / ___

Date Collected: ___ / ___ / ___

Time Collected: _____

Frequency: _____

Ordering Physician: _____

Address: _____

Phone#: _____

Fax#: _____

Insurance Name _____   I.D.#

INFORMATION: INSURANCE

Fasting:
☐ Yes
☐ No

STAT:
☐

CODES

INFORMATION: TEST ORDERED

Test	Code		Test	Code		Test	Code		Test	Code
☐ AFP (Tumor Marker)	SST		☐ Creatinine Urine	U		☐ Lead	RLB		☐ Theophylline	R
☐ Albumin (Alb)	SST		☐ Creatinine Kinase	SST		☐ LH	SST		☐ Thyroglobulin	SST
☐ Alkaline Phosphatase (ALP)	SST		☐ dsDNA Autoantibodies	SST		☐ Lipase	SST		☐ TIBC	SST
☐ ALT (SGPT)	SST		☐ DHEA-SO4	SST		☐ Lipid Profile	SST		☐ Total Protein Serum	SST
☐ Ammonia, Plasma	L		☐ Digoxin	R		☐ Lyme Screen IgG	SST		☐ Total Protein Urine	U
☐ Amylase Serum	SST		☐ EBV VCA IgM	SST		☐ Magnesium Serum	SST		☐ Transferrin	SST
☐ ANA Screen	SST		☐ EBV VCA IgG	SST		☐ Magnesium Urine	U		☐ Triglycerides (Trig)	SST
☐ ANA Profile	SST		☐ EBV Early Antigen	SST		☐ Microalbumin Urine	U		☐ TSH (High Sensitivity)	SST
☐ Anti-TPO Ab	SST		☐ EBV Nuclear Antigen	SST		☐ Microalbumin/Creatinine ratio	U		☐ Uric Acid Serum	SST
☐ Anti-TG Ab	SST		☐ Electrolyte Panel	SST		☐ MMR + V IgG	SST		☐ Uric Acid Urine	U
☐ Apolipoprotein A1	SST		☐ ESR or Sedimentation Rate	L		☐ Non-GYN Cytology, Urine	U		☐ Urinalysis Complete (dipstick and microscopic)	U
☐ Apolipoprotein B	SST		☐ Estradiol	SST		☐ Occult Blood, Feces	FECE!			
☐ AST (SGOT)	SST		☐ Fasting Blood Sugar	GR		☐ Phenobarbital	R		☐ Valproic Acid	R
☐ ASO	SST		☐ Ferritin	SST		☐ Phenytoin or Dilantin	R		☐ Vitamin B12	SST
☐ Basic Metabolic Panel	SST		☐ Folate	SST		☐ Phosphorus Urine	U		☐ Vitamin D, 25 Hydroxy	SST
☐ Beta HCG - Serum	SST		☐ Fructosamine	SST		☐ Phosphorus Serum	SST			
☐ Bilirubin Direct (Dbili)	SST		☐ FSH	SST		☐ PLAC*	SST			
☐ Bilirubin Total (Tbili)	SST		☐ GGT	SST		☐ Potassium (K)	SST			
☐ BNP	L		☐ Glucose Serum	SST		☐ Potassium, Plasma	Gree:		**ADDITIONAL TEST**	
☐ BUN / Creatinine Ratio	SST		☐ Glucose Urine	U		☐ Progesterone Total	SST			
☐ BUN (Urea Nitrogen) S	SST		☐ Glyco Hgb A1c	L		☐ Prolactin	SST		☐ Allergy Complete Food and Respiratory Profile (104 Specific Allergens)	2SST
☐ BUN (Urea Nitrogen) U	U		☐ HDL	SST		☐ Prostatic Acid Phosphatase	SST		☐ Anemia Screen	L, SST
☐ Complement C3	SST		☐ H.Pylori IgG	SST		☐ PSA Free	SST		☐ Cardiac Risk Panel I	L, SST
☐ Complement C4	SST		☐ Hemoglobin/Hematocrit	L		☐ PSA Total	SST		☐ Cardiac Risk Panel II	L, 2SST
☐ CA 15.3	SST		☐ Hepatic Function Panel	SST		☐ PT/INR	B		☐ Diabetic Screen	SST, L
☐ CA - 19.9	SST		☐ Hepatitis A IgM Ab	SST		☐ PTH	SST		☐ Drug Screen with/without ethanol	U
☐ CA - 125	SST		☐ Hepatitis A Total Ab	SST		☐ PTT	B		☐ Epstein-Barr Virus Screen	L, SST
☐ Calcium Serum	SST		☐ Hepatitis B Core IgM Ab	SST		☐ Renal Panel	SST		☐ Female Health Screen I	1L, 3SST, 1UC
☐ Calcium Urine	U		☐ Hepatitis B Core Total	SST		☐ Reticulocyte Count	L		☐ Female Hormone Screen	2SST
☐ Carbamazepine or Tegretol	R		☐ Hepatitis Bs Ab	SST		☐ Rheumatoid Factor	SST		☐ Female Weight Loss Panel	2SST, 1LT, 1UC
☐ Cardio C- Reactive Protein	SST		☐ Hepatitis Bs Ag	SST		☐ RPR (VDRL)	SST			
☐ CBC (w/diff & platelet count)	L		☐ Hepatitis C Total Ab	SST		☐ Sci-70 IgG Autoantibodies	SST		☐ Health Screen II	1L, 2SST
☐ CEA	SST		☐ HSV Type I IgG	SST		☐ SHBG	SST		☐ Heavy Metals	(see back)
☐ Centromere B	SST		☐ HSV Type II IgG	SST		☐ SmRNP IgG Autoantibodies	SST		☐ Hepatitis Screen	SST
☐ Chloride	SST		☐ *HIV 1/2	SST		☐ Sodium (Na)	SST		☐ Male Health Screen I	1L, 3SST, 1UC
☐ Cholesterol	SST		☐ Homocysteine	SST		☐ SS-A & SS-B IgG Autoantibodies	SST		☐ Male Hormone Screen	2SST
☐ CMV IgG	SST		☐ Immunoglobulin E total	SST		☐ T3 Free	SST		☐ Male Weight Loss Panel	2SST, 1LT, 1UC
☐ CO2	SST		☐ Immunoglobulins A, M, G	SST		☐ T3 Total	SST			
☐ Comp Metabolic Panel	SST		☐ Insulin	SST		☐ T3 Uptake	SST		☐ Rheumatic Evaluation	L, 2SST
☐ Cortisol	SST		☐ Iron	SST		☐ T4 Free	SST		☐ Thyroid Antibodies	SST
☐ C-Peptide	SST		☐ Jo-1 Autoantibodies	SST		☐ T4 Total - Thyroxine	SST		☐ Thyroid Comp Screen	SST
☐ C-Reactive Protein (CRP)	SST		☐ LDH	SST		☐ TBG	SST			
☐ Creatinine with eGFR	SST		☐ LDL Direct	SST		☐ Testosterone Total	SST			

Physician Signature _____   DATE ___ / ___ / ___

APPENDIX F: PHLEBOTOMY LOG SHEET

Student's Name: _____

Facility Name: _____

Supervisor's Name: _____

1. Type of Stick		Successful	Unsuccessful	Supervisor Initials
Venipuncture	Dermal Puncture			Date: / /
2. Type of Stick		Successful	Unsuccessful	Supervisor Initials
Venipuncture	Dermal Puncture			Date: / /
3. Type of Stick		Successful	Unsuccessful	Supervisor Initials
Venipuncture	Dermal Puncture			Date: / /
4. Type of Stick		Successful	Unsuccessful	Supervisor Initials
Venipuncture	Dermal Puncture			Date: / /
5. Type of Stick		Successful	Unsuccessful	Supervisor Initials
Venipuncture	Dermal Puncture			Date: / /
6. Type of Stick		Successful	Unsuccessful	Supervisor Initials
Venipuncture	Dermal Puncture			Date: / /
7. Type of Stick		Successful	Unsuccessful	Supervisor Initials
Venipuncture	Dermal Puncture			Date: / /
8. Type of Stick		Successful	Unsuccessful	Supervisor Initials
Venipuncture	Dermal Puncture			Date: / /
9. Type of Stick		Successful	Unsuccessful	Supervisor Initials
Venipuncture	Dermal Puncture			Date: / /

Total Successful Venipuncture _____ / page

Total Successful Dermal Puncture _____ / page

Check sign in appropriate boxes	✓

APPENDIX G: PHLEBOTOMY PROCEDURE SKILLS

COMPETENCY CHECKLIST 5.2: BLEEDING TIME COMPETENCY	1st Attempt	2nd Attempt	3rd Attempt	4th Attempt	5th Attempt	6th Attempt	7th Attempt	8th Attempt	9th Attempt	10th Attempt
1. Verifying Physician's Order.										
2. Greeting, identifying yourself, & identifying the patient (full name & date of birth).										
3. Assembling equipment and supplies.										
4. Washing hands/donning PPE.										
5. Explaining procedure to the patient.										
6. Positioning patient comfortably.										
7. Checking to review if the patient is on medication or dietary restrictions.										
8. Selecting incision site.										
9. Disinfecting site with isopropyl alcohol.										
10. Applying blood pressure cuff.										
11. Positioning the device onto the palmar surface of the forearm.										
12. Blotting blood at 30-second intervals until bleeding stops.										
13. Removing blood pressure cuff.										
14. Applying bandage on the incision site.										
15. Disposing of sharps into a sharps container.										
16. Removing gloves using the proper technique of glove removal.										
17. Disposing of gloves and other supplies into their appropriate containers.										
18. Washing hands using the proper technique of hand washing.										
19. Documenting the procedure electronically or manually.										

COMPETENCY CHECKLIST 5.3: GLUCOSE TESTING COMPETENCY	1st Attempt	2nd Attempt	3rd Attempt	4th Attempt	5th Attempt	6th Attempt	7th Attempt	8th Attempt	9th Attempt	10th Attempt
1. Verifying Physician's Order.										
2. Greeting, identifying yourself, & identifying the patient (full name & date of birth).										
3. Assembling equipment and supplies.										
4. Washing hands/donning PPE.										
5. Explaining procedure to the patient.										
6. Positioning patient comfortably.										
7. Checking to review if the patient is on medication or dietary restrictions.										
8. Selecting incision site.										
9. Disinfecting site with isopropyl alcohol.										
10. Uncapping the reagent strip container.										
11. Positioning the device onto the selected finger.										
12. Placing blood onto the reagent strip.										
13. Applying bandage on the incision site.										
14. Reading results from the blood glucose device.										
15. Cleaning the blood glucose device.										
16. Removing gloves using the proper technique of glove removal.										
17. Disposing of gloves and other supplies into their appropriate containers.										
18. Washing hands using the proper technique of hand washing.										
19. Documenting the procedure electronically or manually.										

COMPETENCY CHECKLIST 5.4: CAPILLARY TUBE BLOOD COLLECTION PROCEDURE	1st Attempt	2nd Attempt	3rd Attempt	4th Attempt	5th Attempt	6th Attempt	7th Attempt	8th Attempt	9th Attempt	10th Attempt
1. Verifying Physician's Order.										
2. Greeting, identifying yourself, & identifying the patient (full name & date of birth).										
3. Assembling equipment and supplies.										
4. Washing hands/donning PPE.										
5. Explaining procedure to the patient.										
6. Positioning patient comfortably.										
7. Checking to review if the patient is on medication or dietary restrictions.										
8. Selecting incision site.										
9. Disinfecting site with isopropyl alcohol.										
10. Positioning the device onto the selected finger.										
11. Wiping the first drop of blood and obtaining blood using a capillary tube.										
12. Sealing of capillary tube on filling the capillary tube using a clay sealant.										
13. Applying bandage on the incision site.										
14. Removing gloves using the proper technique of glove removal.										
15. Disposing of gloves and other supplies into their appropriate containers.										
16. Washing hands using the proper technique of hand washing.										
17. Documenting the procedure electronically or manually.										

COMPETENCY CHECKLIST 5.5: BLOOD SMEAR	1st Attempt	2nd Attempt	3rd Attempt	4th Attempt	5th Attempt	6th Attempt	7th Attempt	8th Attempt	9th Attempt	10th Attempt
1. To create a blood smear, you will need two slides.										
• Sample Slide 1: Blood Sample is placed on it.										
• Slider Slide 2: Used to create a smear with a drop of blood.										
2. Place the sample slide on a flat surface. Handle slides by edges only.										
3. Place a tiny drop of blood near the end of the sample slide.										
4. Place the end (edge) of the slider slide on the drop of the blood so that the blood spreads onto the edges of the slide.										
5. Holding the slider slide at an angle of 45 degrees, push the slider slide in a forward direction creating a smear.										

COMPETENCY CHECKLIST 5.6: VENIPUNCTURE USING A MULTISAMPLE NEEDLE METHOD	1st Attempt	2nd Attempt	3rd Attempt	4th Attempt	5th Attempt	6th Attempt	7th Attempt	8th Attempt	9th Attempt	10th Attempt
1. Verifying Physician's Order.										
2. Greeting, identifying yourself, & identifying the patient (full name & date of birth).										
3. Assembling equipment and supplies.										
4. Washing hands/donning PPE.										
5. Explaining procedure to the patient.										
6. Positioning patient comfortably.										
7. Checking to review if the patient is on medication or dietary restrictions.										
8. Applying tourniquet at the appropriate location.										
9. Selecting incision site.										
10. Removing tourniquet.										
11. Disinfecting site with isopropyl alcohol.										
12. Connecting needle to needle collection holder, inspect needle (use appropriate gauge needle).										

13. Reapplying tourniquet.											
14. With the fingers (thumb or forefinger) of the non-needle unit carrying hand, pulling the skin taut below the site of the puncture.											
15. With the needle unit carrying hand, inserting the needle at an appropriate angle.											
16. Releasing the tourniquet when the blood starts to fill the initial tube.											
17. Removing the final tube from the evacuated tube holder prior to removing the needle.											
18. Removing the needle and turning on (initiating) the safety device.											
19. Applying direct pressure on incision site with a 2x2 gauze pad.											
20. Disposing of sharps into a sharps container.											
21. Mixing tubes (follow the correct number of inversions).											
22. Blood collection tube labeling must be performed as per the facility policy.											
23. Checking on the patient for hemostasis by inspecting the site of the puncture.											
24. Applying bandage once the bleeding stops.											
25. Packaging specimen for transport.											
26. Removing gloves using the proper technique of glove removal.											
27. Disposing of gloves and other supplies into their appropriate containers.											
28. Washing hands using the proper technique of hand washing.											
29. Documenting the procedure electronically or manually.											

COMPETENCY CHECKLIST 5.7: VENIPUNCTURE USING A WINGED INFUSION OR BUTTERFLY NEEDLE METHOD	1st Attempt	2nd Attempt	3rd Attempt	4th Attempt	5th Attempt	6th Attempt	7th Attempt	8th Attempt	9th Attempt	10th Attempt
1. Verifying Physician's Order.										
2. Greeting, identifying yourself, & identifying the patient (full name & date of birth).										
3. Assembling equipment and supplies.										
4. Washing hands/donning PPE.										
5. Explaining procedure to the patient.										
6. Positioning patient comfortably.										
7. Checking to review if the patient is on medication or dietary restrictions.										
8. Applying tourniquet at the appropriate location.										
9. Selecting incision site.										
10. Removing tourniquet.										
11. Disinfecting site with isopropyl alcohol.										
12. Connecting butterfly needle to needle collection holder, inspect needle (use appropriate gauge needle).										
13. Reapplying tourniquet.										
14. With the butterfly needle unit carrying hand, inserting the needle at an appropriate angle.										
15. Releasing the tourniquet when the blood starts to fill the initial tube.										
16. Removing the final tube from the evacuated tube holder prior to removing the needle.										
17. Removing the needle and turning on (initiating) the safety device.										
18. Applying direct pressure on incision site with a 2x2 gauze pad.										
19. Disposing of sharps into a sharps container.										
20. Mixing tubes (follow the correct number of inversions).										
21. Blood collection tube labeling must be performed as per the facility policy.										

	1st Attempt	2nd Attempt	3rd Attempt	4th Attempt	5th Attempt	6th Attempt	7th Attempt	8th Attempt	9th Attempt	10th Attempt
22. Checking on the patient for hemostasis by inspecting the site of the puncture.										
23. Applying bandage once the bleeding stops.										
24. Packaging specimen for transport.										
25. Removing gloves using the proper technique of glove removal.										
26. Disposing of gloves and other supplies into their appropriate containers.										
27. Washing hands using the proper technique of hand washing.										
28. Documenting the procedure electronically or manually.										

COMPETENCY CHECKLIST 5.8: VENIPUNCTURE USING A SYRINGE AND NEEDLE (METHOD)	1st Attempt	2nd Attempt	3rd Attempt	4th Attempt	5th Attempt	6th Attempt	7th Attempt	8th Attempt	9th Attempt	10th Attempt
1 Verifying Physician's Order.										
2 Greeting, identifying yourself, & identifying the patient (full name & date of birth).										
3 Assembling equipment and supplies.										
4 Washing hands/donning PPE.										
5. Explaining procedure to the patient.										
6. Positioning patient comfortably.										
7. Checking to review if the patient is on medication or dietary restrictions.										
8. Applying tourniquet at the appropriate location.										
9. Selecting incision site.										
10. Removing tourniquet.										
11. Disinfecting site with isopropyl alcohol.										
12. Connecting needle to the syringe, inspecting needle (use appropriate gauge needle).										
13. Reapplying tourniquet.										
14. With the fingers (thumb or forefinger) of the non-needle-syringe unit carrying hand, pulling the skin taut below the site of the puncture.										

15. With the needle-syringe unit carrying hand, inserting the needle at an appropriate angle.											
16. Releasing the tourniquet.											
17. Removing the needle.											
18. Applying direct pressure on incision site with a 2x2 gauze pad.											
19. Using a transfer device. The blood from the syringe is transferred into the evacuated tube.											
20. Disposing of sharps into a sharps container.											
21. Mixing tube (follow the correct number of inversions).											
22. Blood collection tube labeling must be performed as per the facility policy.											
23. Checking on the patient for hemostasis by inspecting the site of the puncture.											
24. Applying bandage once the bleeding stops.											
25. Packaging specimen for transport.											
26. Removing gloves using the proper technique of glove removal.											
27. Disposing of gloves and other supplies into their appropriate containers.											
28. Washing hands using the proper technique of hand washing.											
29. Documenting the procedure electronically or manually.											

PRACTICE EXAM 1

1. Which of the following is not the duty of the phlebotomy technician:
a. Performing proper patient identification for appropriate labeling.
b. Assembling, maintaining and keeping track of inventory for equipment and supplies required to perform the phlebotomy procedure.
c. Preparing the patient for the procedure.
d. Interpreting the results of the venipuncture procedures performed.

2. The abbreviation OSHA stands for:
a. Occupational Safety and Health Administration
b. Occupational Safety and Health Act
c. Occupational Safety and Hazard Administration
d. Occupational Safety and Health Association

3. Healthcare safety hazards includes all of the following except:
a. Biological Hazards
b. Sharps Hazard
c. Financial Hazards
d. Chemical Hazards

4. Procedure to follow post–exposure to blood

a.	Document the injury.
b.	The employer must provide medical evaluation and follow-up.
c.	Wash the area with water or antiseptic.
d.	Report to the employer.

Sequence the procedure.
a. C, D, A, B
b. A, B, C, D
c. B, C, A, D
d. D, A, C, B

5. A process that begins when an agent leaves its reservoir or host through a portal of exit, then is conveyed by some mode of transmission and enters through an appropriate portal of entry to infect a susceptible host.
a. Latex allergy
b. Chain of infection
c. Contact Dermatitis
d. Physical Hazard

6. The precautions that apply to patients with draining wound:
a. Contact Precautions
b. Droplet Precautions
c. Airborne Precautions
d. None of the Options

7. The precautions that apply to patients with pressure ulcers:
a. Contact Precautions
b. Droplet Precautions
c. Airborne Precautions
d. None of the Options

8. The precautions that apply to patients with draining body fluids:
a. Contact Precautions
b. Droplet Precautions
c. Airborne Precautions
d. None of the Options

9. The precautions that apply to patients with ostomy tubes:
a. Contact Precautions
b. Droplet Precautions
c. Airborne Precautions
d. None of the Options

10. The precautions that apply to patients with respiratory viruses:
a. Contact Precautions
b. Droplet Precautions
c. Airborne Precautions
d. None of the Options

11. The precautions that apply to patients with Bordetella pertussis.
a. Contact Precautions
b. Droplet Precautions
c. Airborne Precautions
d. None of the Options

12. The precautions that apply to patients with Tuberculosis.
a. Contact Precautions

b. Droplet Precautions
c. Airborne Precautions
d. None of the Options

13. The precautions that apply to patients with Measles.
a. Contact Precautions
b. Droplet Precautions
c. Airborne Precautions
d. None of the Options

14. Breaking the chain of infection can be done by performing all the following.

a.	Using effective hand hygiene.
b.	Using personal protective equipment (PPE).
c.	Isolating patients with infectious diseases.
d.	Follow standard precautions.
e.	None of the options (a, b, c, d)
f.	All of the options above (a, b, c, d, e)

a. A, B, C, D
b. E
c. A, B, C
d. F

15. The proper technique of hand washing involves applying soap and rubbing the hands for at least
a. 60 seconds
b. 2 minutes
c. 15 seconds
d. 5 minutes

16. The abbreviation PPE stands for:
a. Professional protective equipment
b. Personal protective equipment
c. Professional protective essentials
d. Personal protective equipment

17. Given the following PPE, the correct PPE donning order would be:

a.	Gloves
b.	Goggles or face shield
c.	Gown
d.	Mask or respirator

Sequence the procedure.
a. C, D, B, A
b. A, B, C, D

c. B, C, A, D
d. D, A, C, B

18. Given the following PPE, the correct order of removing PPE would be:

a.	Mask or respirator
b.	Gown
c.	Goggles or face shield
d.	Gloves

Sequence the procedure.
a. C, D, B, A
b. A, B, C, D
c. B, C, A, D
d. D, C, B, A

19. _____ is a process that destroys or eliminates all forms of microbial life and can be carried out via physical or chemical methods.
a. Sterilization
b. Disinfection
c. Cleaning
d. None of the options

20. _____ is a process that eliminates many or all pathogenic microorganisms, except some bacterial spores.
a. Sterilization
b. Disinfection
c. Cleaning
d. None of the options

21. _____ is the process of removing visible soil from objects and surfaces.
a. Sterilization
b. Disinfection
c. Cleaning
d. None of the options

22. Threatening or causing bodily injury to another person, it may be a crime or a tort.
a. Assault
b. Battery
c. Defamation
d. Libel

23. Touching a patient without his or her consent is termed as a battery, it can either be a civil or criminal offense.
a. Malpractice
b. Battery
c. Defamation
d. Libel

24. In general is a written or oral statement which causes harm to the reputation of a person or third party.
a. Malpractice
b. Battery
c. Defamation
d. Libel

25. A defamatory statement presented in an oral or spoken format.
a. Slander
b. Battery
c. Defamation
d. Libel

26. A defamatory statement presented in a published or written format.
a. Malpractice
b. Battery
c. Defamation
d. Libel

27. Intentionally hiding the truth for unlawful gains.
a. Assault
b. Fraud
c. Defamation
d. Libel

28. A substandard delivery of care by the healthcare provider causing injury to the patient.
a. Malpractice
b. Battery
c. Defamation
d. Libel

29. HIPAA stands for:
a. Health Insurance Portability and Administration Act
b. Health Information Portability and Accountability Act

c. Health Insurance Portability and Accountability Administration
d. Health Insurance Portability and Accountability Act

30. A process in which the permission is granted from the patient prior to the start of a healthcare procedure.
a. Informed Consent
b. Expressed Consent
c. Implied Consent
d. None of the options

31. A type of consent in which the person expresses the permission in written or spoken words before the onset of a healthcare procedure.
a. Informed Consent
b. Expressed Consent
c. Implied Consent
d. None of the options

32. A type of consent in which the permission is not expressed but rather inferred by the person's action, signs, and facts.
a. Informed Consent
b. Expressed Consent
c. Implied Consent:
d. None of the options

33. Basic elements of negligence includes all of the following except:
a. Duty
b. Breach of duty
c. Standard of care
d. Direct cause
e. Damage

34. Employers are liable for the actions of an employee within the course and scope of their employment.
a. Res ipsa Loquitor
b. Respondeat Superior
c. Abandonment
d. Scope of Practice

35. Connective tissue has the following characteristic(s):
a. Ground Substance
b. Fibers
c. Cells
d. All of the options

36. Red blood cells are also known as:

a. Erythrocytes

b. Leukocytes

c. Lymphocytes

d. Thrombocytes

37. White blood cells are also known as:

a. Erythrocytes

b. Leukocytes

c. Lymphocytes

d. Thrombocytes

38. Platelets are also known as:

a. Erythrocytes

b. Leukocytes

c. Lymphocytes

d. Thrombocytes

39. The plasma portion of the blood is about

a. 55%

b. 70%

c. 45%

d. 20%

40. The formed element portion of the blood is about

a. 55%

b. 70%

c. 45%

d. 20%

41. The formed elements consists of all of the following except:

a. Erythrocytes

b. Leukocytes

c. Thrombocytes

d. Plasma

42. The white blood cells includes all of the following except:

a. Basophils

b. Eosinophils

c. Thrombocytes

d. Neutrophils

e. Monocytes

f. Lymphocytes

43. When leukocytes increase in number, the condition is termed as

a. Eosinophilia

b. Leukocytosis

c. Neutrophilia

d. Basophilia

44. When leukocytes decrease in number, the condition is termed as

a. Neutropenia

b. Monocytopenia

c. Leukopenia

d. Lymphocytopenia

45. The white blood cells that are granulocytes are all of the following except:

a. Eosinophils

b. Basophils

c. Monocytes

d. Neutrophils

46. The white blood cell that is agranulocytes:

a. Basophils

b. Eosinophils

c. Neutrophils

d. Monocytes

47. Releases heparin and histamine. Heparin inhibits coagulation (clotting) making it possible for the other white blood cells to flow and Histamine cause vasodilation for increasing the blood flow to the area.

a. Basophils

b. Eosinophils

c. Neutrophils

d. Monocytes

e. Lymphocytes

48. Provide immune response against parasitic infection. They are also seen in response to an allergic reaction.

a. Basophils

b. Eosinophils

c. Neutrophils

d. Monocytes

e. Lymphocytes

49. Provides immunity by protecting the body against
bacteria and fungi. They are phagocytic in nature.

a. Basophils
b. Eosinophils
c. Neutrophils
d. Monocytes
e. Lymphocytes

50. Performs the function of phagocytes by the process of
phagocytosis, however, they are less phagocytic in
nature than the neutrophils. They help other white
blood cells in recognizing the pathogens.

a. Basophils
b. Eosinophils
c. Neutrophils
d. Monocytes
e. Lymphocytes

PRACTICE EXAM 1: ANSWER SHEET

TOTAL SCORE: 50 **YOUR SCORE:** _____

1.	2.	3.	4.	5.	6.	7.	8.	9.	10.
11.	12.	13.	14.	15.	16.	17.	18.	19.	20.
21.	22.	23.	24.	25.	26.	27.	28.	29.	30.
31.	32.	33.	34.	35.	36.	37.	38.	39.	40.
41.	42.	43.	44.	45.	46.	47.	48.	49.	50.

PRACTICE EXAM 2

1. They are of 3 types: T cells, B cells, and Natural killer cells.
   a. Basophils
   b. Eosinophils
   c. Neutrophils
   d. Monocytes
   e. Lymphocytes

2. Process of Phagocytosis

a.	The antigen enters the phagocytic cell, after which the antigen is engulfed forming a phagosome. The phagosome and lysosome form phagolysosome.
b.	Remains of the digestion process are expelled out of the cell in the form of debris.
c.	The antigen coming in contact with the phagocytic cell.
d.	Phagocyte-antigen adherence takes place.
e.	Digestion of the antigen.

Sequence the procedure.
   a. A, B, C, D, E
   b. C, D, A, E, B
   c. B, C, A, D, E
   d. D, C, E, A, B

3. Following are the steps taken to obtain:
   Collect Blood in the blood collection tube, Clot blood for 30-45 minutes, Centrifuge for 15 minutes.
   a. To obtain a plasma sample
   b. To obtain a whole blood sample
   c. To obtain a serum sample
   d. None of the following

4. Following are the steps taken to obtain:
   Collect Blood in the blood collection tube, Centrifuge for 15 minutes.
   a. To obtain a plasma sample
   b. To obtain a whole blood sample
   c. To obtain a serum sample
   d. None of the following

5. Antigens are substances that are produced in the body in response to an invading micro-organism.
   a. True
   b. False

6. Antibodies on entering the body activate the immune response which leads to the production of an antibody.
   a. True
   b. False

7. Immunoglobulins are also known as antigens.
   a. True
   b. False

8. Blood transfusion is the procedure of transferring blood from the donor to the recipient.
   a. True
   b. False

9. The arterial system consists of all of the following except:
   a. Aorta
   b. Arteries
   c. Capillaries
   d. Arterioles

10. The venous system consists of all of the following except:
    a. Vena cava
    b. Venule
    c. Vein
    d. Capillaries

11. The main function is to give oxygen and nutrient to the tissues and collect carbon dioxide and waste from the tissues.
    a. Vein
    b. Capillaries
    c. Arteries
    d. None of the options.

12. Carries deoxygenated blood from the body to the heart.
    a. Vein
    b. Capillaries
    c. Arteries
    d. None of the options.

13. Carries oxygenated blood (oxygen-rich blood) from the heart to the body.
a. Vein
b. Capillaries
c. Arteries
d. None of the options.

14. Vasodilation refers to the increase in diameter of the blood vessels.
a. True
b. False

15. Vasoconstriction refers to the decrease in diameter of the blood vessels.
a. True
b. False

16. The middle layer of the skin is called the
a. Hypodermis
b. Dermis
c. Epidermis
d. Subcutaneous layer

17. The inner layer of the skin is called the
a. Hypodermis
b. Dermis
c. Subcutaneous layer
d. Epidermis

18. The outer layer of the skin is called the
a. Hypodermis
b. Dermis
c. Epidermis
d. None of the options.

19. Receives deoxygenated blood from superior and inferior vena cava.
a. Right Atrium
b. Right Ventricle
c. Left Atrium
d. Left Ventricle

20. Receives oxygenated blood from both (right and left) lungs via the pulmonary vein.
a. Right Atrium
b. Right Ventricle
c. Left Atrium

d. Left Ventricle

21. Receives the deoxygenated blood from right atrium via the tricuspid valve and pumps it out of the heart via the pulmonary artery to the right and the left lung.
a. Right Atrium
b. Right Ventricle
c. Left Atrium
d. Left Ventricle

22. Receives oxygenated blood from left atrium via the bicuspid valve and pumps it out of the heart to the rest of the body via the aorta.
a. Right Atrium
b. Right Ventricle
c. Left Atrium
d. Left Ventricle

23. The respiratory system is also known as the integumentary system of the human body.
a. True
b. False

24. Exhalation is a process through which carbon dioxide is exhaled out of the lungs through the nose.
a. True
b. False

25. Inhalation is a process through which oxygen is inhaled into the lungs through the nose.
a. True
b. False

26. The bones of the LEG and FOOT includes all of the following except:
a. Femur
b. Patella
c. Pelvis
d. Tibia
e. Fibula

27. The bones of the ARM and HAND includes all of the following except:
a. Humerus
b. Ulna
c. Clavicle
d. Radius

e. Carpals

28. Which of the following in not the bone of the axial skeleton system
a. Skull
b. Spinal Column
c. Sacrum
d. Scapula
e. Sternum

29. Which of the following is not the bone of the appendicular skeleton system?
a. Femur
b. Patella
c. Metacarpals
d. Tibia
e. Fibula

30. The spinal cord carries and transfers signal between the brain and the rest of the body.
a. True
b. False

31. _____ are present in a pair, two in number. They play a vital role in the urinary system. They are present in the back (abdominal region) and are bean shaped.
a. Kidneys
b. Ureters
c. Urinary bladder
d. Urethra

32. _____ are tubes that carry urine from the kidney to the urinary bladder.
a. Kidneys
b. Ureters
c. Urinary bladder
d. Urethra

33. _____ is a bag or sac that is located in the lower abdominal region. The main function of the bladder is to hold the urine until it is expelled out via the urethra.
a. Kidneys
b. Ureters
c. Urinary bladder
d. Urethra

34. The _____ is the structure through which the urine is expelled out of the urinary bladder. It serves as a passage for passing the urine from (out of the) the bladder to the out of the human body.
a. Kidneys
b. Ureters
c. Urinary bladder
d. Urethra

35. The _____ are the structural working units of the kidney.
a. Kidneys
b. Nephron
c. Ureters
d. Urinary bladder

36. Coronal Plane or Frontal Plane divides the human body into front and back.
a. True
b. False

37. Sagittal Plane or Median Plane divides the human body into left & right.
a. True
b. False

38. Transverse Plane or Horizontal Plane divides the human body into upper and lower parts.
a. True
b. False

39. Dorsal/Posterior: Front of the body.
a. True
b. False

40. Ventral/Anterior: Back of the body.
a. True
b. False

41. Lateral: Towards the center of the body.
a. True
b. False

42. Medial: Towards the side
    a. True
    b. False

43. Distal: Away from a point of reference
    a. True
    b. False

44. Proximal: Towards a point of reference
    a. True
    b. False

45. ROOT: Gives meaning to the medical term
    a. True
    b. False

46. SUFFIX: This part is the one with which the medical term may end
    a. True
    b. False

47. PREFIX: This part is the one with which the medical term may start
    a. Truc
    b. False

48. COMBINING VOWEL: Is what combines a root to another root, a root to a suffix. (a, e, i, o, u)
    a. True
    b. False

49. The affix a or an means with
    a. True
    b. False

50. The affix ab means away from
    a. True
    b. False

PRACTICE EXAM 2: ANSWER SHEET

TOTAL SCORE: <u>50</u>   YOUR SCORE: _____

1.	2.	3.	4.	5.	6.	7.	8.	9.	10.
11.	12.	13.	14.	15.	16.	17.	18.	19.	20.
21.	22.	23.	24.	25.	26.	27.	28.	29.	30.
31.	32.	33.	34.	35.	36.	37.	38.	39.	40.
41.	42.	43.	44.	45.	46.	47.	48.	49.	50.

PRACTICE EXAM 3

1. The affix ad means towards
   a. True
   b. False

2. The affix adipo means fat
   a. True
   b. False

3. The affix -al means related to
   a. True
   b. False

4. The affix -algia means breathing difficulty
   a. True
   b. False

5. The affix angio means vessel
   a. True
   b. False

6. The affix ante means towards front
   a. True
   b. False

7. The affix arter means vein
   a. True
   b. False

8. The affix aspir means removal
   a. True
   b. False

9. The affix axill means armpit
   a. True
   b. False

10. The affix bacteri means bacteria
    a. True
    b. False

11. The affix baro means measure
    a. True
    b. False

12. The affix brachi means artery
    a. True
    b. False

13. The affix brady means fast
    a. True
    b. False

14. The affix bi means two
    a. True
    b. False

15. The affix cardio means heart
    a. True
    b. False

16. The affix -cardium means heart
    a. True
    b. False

17. The affix carp means carpal bones
    a. True
    b. False

18. The affix -cephalic means head
    a. True
    b. False

19. The affix cephalo means head
    a. True
    b. False

20. The affix chondro means cartilage
    a. True
    b. False

21. The affix -cidal means killing in nature
    a. True
    b. False

22. The affix -clast means break into fragments
    a. True
    b. False

23. The affix contra means opposite or against
    a. True
    b. False

24. The affix costo means rib
    a. True
    b. False

25. The affix -constrict means narrowing
    a. True
    b. False

26. The affix cryo means hot
    a. True
    b. False

27. The affix cutane means skin
    a. True
    b. False

28. The affix cyano means red color
    a. True
    b. False

29. The affix cysto means urinary bladder
    a. True
    b. False

30. The affix -cytes means cell
    a. True
    b. False

31. The affix cyto means cell
    a. True
    b. False

32. The affix dermato means skin
    a. True
    b. False

33. The affix dors means back or behind
    a. True
    b. False

34. The affix -dynia means difficulty
    a. True
    b. False

35. The affix dys means difficult
    a. True
    b. False

36. The affix -eal means related to
    a. True
    b. False

37. The affix -ectomy means surgical removal of a body part
    a. True
    b. False

38. The affix -emesis means vomit
    a. True
    b. False

39. The affix encephalo means nerves
    a. True
    b. False

40. The affix endo means internal
    a. True
    b. False

41. The affix epi means above or upon
    a. True
    b. False

42. The affix erythr means white
    a. True
    b. False

43. The affix esthesi means sensation
    a. True
    b. False

44. The affix ex means outer
    a. True
    b. False

45. The affix fossa means hollow area
    a. True
    b. False

46. The affix -gram means recording
    a. True
    b. False

47. The affix -graph means generating the recording
    a. True
    b. False

48. The affix -graphy means recording process
    a. True
    b. False

49. The affix hemat means blood
    a. True
    b. False

50. The affix hemo means blood
    a. True
    b. False

PRACTICE EXAM 3: ANSWER SHEET

TOTAL SCORE: <u>50</u>   YOUR SCORE: _____

1.	2.	3.	4.	5.	6.	7.	8.	9.	10.
11.	12.	13.	14.	15.	16.	17.	18.	19.	20.
21.	22.	23.	24.	25.	26.	27.	28.	29.	30.
31.	32.	33.	34.	35.	36.	37.	38.	39.	40.
41.	42.	43.	44.	45.	46.	47.	48.	49.	50.

PRACTICE EXAM 4

1. The affix hemi means complete
   a. True
   b. False

2. The affix hepat means liver
   a. True
   b. False

3. The affix histo means tissue
   a. True
   b. False

4. The affix hyper means extreme or beyond
   a. True
   b. False

5. The affix hypo means below or under
   a. True
   b. False

6. The affix infra means beneath or below
   a. True
   b. False

7. The affix inter means between
   a. True
   b. False

8. The affix intra means within
   a. True
   b. False

9. The affix iso means different
   a. True
   b. False

10. The affix -itis means inflammation
    a. True
    b. False

11. The affix leuko means red
    a. True
    b. False

12. The affix levo or laevo means left
    a. True
    b. False

13. The affix lipo means fat
    a. True
    b. False

14. The affix -logy means study of
    a. True
    b. False

15. The affix -lysis means destruction
    a. True
    b. False

16. The affix -metry means measure
    a. True
    b. False

17. The affix myco means muscles
    a. True
    b. False

18. The affix naso means nose
    a. True
    b. False

19. The affix neo means old
    a. True
    b. False

20. The affix nephro means related to nervous system
    a. True
    b. False

21. The affix nocti means day
    a. True
    b. False

22. The affix -oma means tumor
    a. True
    b. False

23. The affix onco means tumor
    a. True
    b. False

24. The affix para means beside
    a. True
    b. False

25. The affix -paresis means strong
    a. True
    b. False

26. The affix patho means disease
    a. True
    b. False

27. The affix -pathy means disorder
    a. True
    b. False

28. The affix -penia means deficiency
    a. True
    b. False

29. The affix peri means surrounding or around
    a. True
    b. False

30. The affix phleb means artery
    a. True
    b. False

31. The affix -plegia means paralysis
    a. True
    b. False

32. The affix pneumo means lungs
    a. True
    b. False

33. The affix -pnea means breathing
    a. True
    b. False

34. The affix -rrhage means flow of discharge
    a. True
    b. False

35. The affix -rrhagia means abnormal flow of discharge
    a. True
    b. False

36. The affix -rrhaphy means suture
    a. True
    b. False

37. The affix -rrhea means discharge
    a. True
    b. False

38. The affix sero means serum
    a. True
    b. False

39. The affix -stasis means slowing or stopping
    a. True
    b. False

40. The affix steno means narrowing
    a. True
    b. False

41. The affix -stomy means a surgical procedure to create an opening.
    a. True
    b. False

42. The affix sub means lower or under
    a. True
    b. False

43. The affix tachy means slow
    a. True
    b. False

44. The affix thrombo means blood clot
    a. True
    b. False

45. The affix -tomy means incision
    a. True
    b. False

46. The affix vaso means vessel
    a. True
    b. False

47. The affix ven means vein
- a. True
- b. False

48. The affix vir means virus
- a. True
- b. False

49. The affix viscero means organ
- a. True
- b. False

50. Steps in wearing gloves:

a.	Perform the procedure.
b.	Don (wear) gloves.
c.	Select proper size gloves.
d.	Perform hand hygiene.

Sequence the procedure.

- a. A, B, C, D
- b. C, D, A, B
- c. B, C, A, D
- d. D, C, B, A

PRACTICE EXAM 4: ANSWER SHEET

TOTAL SCORE: 50   **YOUR SCORE: _____**

1.	2.	3.	4.	5.	6.	7.	8.	9.	10.
11.	12.	13.	14.	15.	16.	17.	18.	19.	20.
21.	22.	23.	24.	25.	26.	27.	28.	29.	30.
31.	32.	33.	34.	35.	36.	37.	38.	39.	40.
41.	42.	43.	44.	45.	46.	47.	48.	49.	50.

PRACTICE EXAM 5

1. Steps in removing gloves:

a.	Post-procedure.
b.	Perform hand hygiene.
c.	Remove gloves.
d.	Discard them into their appropriate container.

Sequence the procedure.
   a. A, B, C, D
   b. C, D, A, B
   c. A, C, D, B
   d. D, C, B, A

2. Gloves should be removed and discarded if
   a. They are soiled with blood,
   b. After contact with patient,
   c. If they are damaged or torn.
   d. All of the options.

3. If the glove is too large, the phlebotomy technician may have difficulty holding the equipment and supplies properly making it difficult to perform the procedure.
   a. True
   b. False

4. Tourniquet is an elastic band like strip that is wrapped or tied around the patient's arm. The main function of the tourniquet in to create pressure and make the vein prominent or visible for venipuncture.
   a. True
   b. False

5. The tourniquet once placed on the patient's arm must be untied/removed within ____ minute. It should not stay in place for more than _____ minute.
   a. 3
   b. 5
   c. 7
   d. 1

6. The tourniquet should not be too tight on the patient's arm, since this may stop the flow of blood to the arm.
   a. True
   b. False

7. When performing venipuncture procedure on the arm, it is recommended that the tourniquet is applied _____ inches above the site of the puncture.
   a. 1-2
   b. 2-6
   c. 3-4
   d. 5-7

8. Post application of the topical alcohol prep pad on the surface of the skin, let the skin air dry before performing the procedure.
   a. True
   b. False

9. If the gauge of the needle is smaller, the lumen of the needle would be smaller.
   a. True
   b. False

10. Lower the number (needle gauge), smaller the needle lumen (diameter).
    a. True
    b. False

11. _____ of the needle is the part of the needle that is sharp and that functions to puncture the skin; it is the first part of the needle that comes in contact with the skin of the puncture site.
    a. Lumen
    b. Bevel
    c. Shaft
    d. Point
    e. Hub

12. _____ is the opening of the needle through which the blood passes through. While performing venipuncture, the bevel of the needle should face up before inserting the needle for drawing blood.
    a. Lumen
    b. Bevel
    c. Point
    d. Hub

13. _____ is the inside space of the tubular structure needle.
    a. Lumen
    b. Bevel
    c. Shaft
    d. Point
    e. Hub

14. _____ is the tubular portion of the needle.
    a. Lumen
    b. Bevel
    c. Point
    d. Shaft
    e. Hub

15. _____ is the end part of the needle. It is usually made up of plastic.
    a. Shaft
    b. Lumen
    c. Bevel
    d. Point
    e. Hub

16. If a small gauge needle that has a larger lumen is used to perform the procedure on a smaller diameter vein, the blood sample collected may become hemolyzed.
    a. True
    b. False

17. If a large gauge needle that has a smaller lumen is used to perform the procedure on a larger diameter vein, the blood sample collected may become clotted.
    a. True
    b. False

18. Angle at which the needle is inserted for blood draws:
    a. 15 degree for a superficial vein.
    b. 45 degree for a superficial vein.
    c. 5 degree for a superficial vein.
    d. 60 degree for a superficial vein.

19. Angle at which the needle is inserted for blood draws:
    a. 10 degree for a deeper vein.
    b. 5 degree for a deeper vein.
    c. 30 degree for a deeper vein.
    d. 60 degree for a deeper vein.

20. Which of the following in not an anticoagulant?
    a. EDTA (Ethylene-diamine-tetra-acetic-acid)
    b. Sodium Citrate
    c. Potassium Oxalate
    d. Thixotropic Gel

21. Which of the following in a clot activator?
    a. Heparin
    b. Sodium Fluoride
    c. Lithium Idoacetate
    d. Silica

22. Which of the following additive can be found in the light green tube?
    a. Lithium Heparin with Gel
    b. Sodium Heparin
    c. Potassium Oxalate
    d. Acid Citrate

23. Which of the following additive can be found in the red tube?
    a. Clot Activator
    b. SPS
    c. Thrombin-Based Clot Activator
    d. Lithium Heparin

24. Which of the following additive can be found in the yellow tube non sterile?
    a. Sodium Heparin
    b. Potassium Oxalate
    c. Acid Citrate Dextrose
    d. Sodium Polyanethol Sulfonate

25. Which of the following additive can be found in the light blue tube?
    a. Sodium Citrate
    b. Sodium Heparin
    c. Potassium Oxalate
    d. Acid Citrate

26. Which of the following additive can be found in the gray tube?
    a. Potassium Oxalate/Sodium Fluoride
    b. Sodium Citrate
    c. Sodium Heparin
    d. Potassium Oxalate

27. Which of the following additive can be found in the gold tube?
    a. Clot activator and gel
    b. Sodium Heparin
    c. Potassium Oxalate
    d. Acid Citrate

28. Which of the following additive can be found in the lavender tube?
    a. EDTA K_2, EDTA K_3
    b. Sodium Citrate
    c. Sodium Heparin
    d. Potassium Oxalate

29. Which of the following additive can be found in the green tube?
    a. Clot activator and gel
    b. Sodium Heparin
    c. Potassium Oxalate
    d. Acid Citrate

30. Which of the following additive can be found in the royal blue tube?
    a. Sodium EDTA
    b. SPS
    c. Thrombin-Based Clot Activator
    d. Lithium Heparin

31. Which of the following additive can be found in the orange tube?
    a. Thrombin-based clot activator
    b. Sodium Heparin
    c. Potassium Oxalate
    d. Acid Citrate

32. Which of the following additive can be found in the tan tube?
    a. K_2EDTA
    b. SPS
    c. Thrombin-Based Clot Activator
    d. Lithium Heparin

33. Which of the following additive can be found in the pink tube?
    a. K_2EDTA
    b. SPS
    c. Thrombin-Based Clot Activator

    d. Lithium Heparin

34. The correct order of draw for venipuncture:
    a. Culture Tubes : Light Blue : Red : Green : Lavender : Gray
    b. Culture Tubes : Light Blue : Green : Red : Lavender : Gray
    c. Culture Tubes : Red: Light Blue : Green : Lavender : Gray
    d. Culture Tubes: Light Blue : Red : Gray : Lavender : Green

35. When performing heel puncture on infants, a warming device is required to warm the area. This is done to increase the flow of blood in the area. Prior to performing the dermal puncture the warming device is placed in contact with the heel for _____ minutes in duration.
    a. 3 to 5
    b. 1 to 3
    c. 10 to 15
    d. 2 to 8

36. When performing heel puncture on an infant, the depth of the puncture should not exceed.
    a. 2.0 mm
    b. 4.0 mm
    c. 3.0 mm
    d. 1.0 mm

37. When performing heel puncture on an infant, the width of the puncture should not exceed.
    a. 2.4 mm
    b. 4.4 mm
    c. 3.4 mm
    d. 1.4 mm

38. The correct order of draw for a dermal puncture:
    a. Lavender : Light Green : Green : Gray : Yellow : Red
    b. Lavender : Gray : Light Green : Green : Yellow : Red
    c. Lavender : Gray : Green : Light Green : Yellow : Red
    d. Lavender : Green : Light Green : Gray : Yellow : Red

39. When performing bleeding time test procedure the blood pressure cuff applied must be inflated to:
    a. 40 mm Hg
    b. 70 mm Hg
    c. 20 mm Hg
    d. 100 mm Hg

40. When performing bleeding time test procedure, the incision site should be the:
    a. Antecubital region
    b. Arm region
    c. Forearm region
    d. Hand region

41. When performing bleeding time test procedure the blood is blotted using a filter paper every:
    a. 30 seconds
    b. 10 seconds
    c. 15 seconds
    d. 60 seconds

42. Small spot on the skin, red or purple in color, caused by hemorrhage to the capillary (blood vessel).
    a. Petechiae
    b. Septicemia
    c. Hematoma
    d. Hemoconcentration

43. Not following the precautions and proper procedural standards such as (using contaminated equipment and supplies may cause infection in the blood.
    a. Petechiae
    b. Septicemia
    c. Hematoma
    d. Hemoconcentration

44. Occurs due to injury caused by the needle insertion leading to accumulation of blood external to the blood vessels and within the tissue causing internal bleeding of the tissue.
    a. Petechiae
    b. Septicemia
    c. Hematoma
    d. Hemoconcentration

45. Increase in concentration of red blood cells and other formed elements.
    a. Petechiae
    b. Septicemia
    c. Hematoma
    d. Hemoconcentration

46. Inflammation of vein may occur due to injury to that vein due to venipuncture or due to blood clot formation.
    a. Thrombophlebitis
    b. Phlebitis
    c. Vasovagal reaction
    d. Compartmental syndrome

47. A blood clot formed within the vein further cause's inflammation, redness, and pain.
    a. Thrombophlebitis
    b. Phlebitis
    c. Vasovagal reaction
    d. Compartmental syndrome

48. A patient may experience this as a result of a shock or pain; it can lead to fainting.
    a. Seizures
    b. Phlebitis
    c. Vasovagal reaction
    d. Syncope

49. A breakdown of red blood cells. Breakdown of RBCs causes the release of hemoglobin.
    a. Septicemia
    b. Hematoma
    c. Hemoconcentration
    d. Hemolysis

50. Requires immediate test results.
    a. STAT
    b. ASAP
    c. ROUTINE
    d. TIMED

PRACTICE EXAM 5: ANSWER SHEET

TOTAL SCORE: 50   **YOUR SCORE: _____**

1.	2.	3.	4.	5.	6.	7.	8.	9.	10.
11.	12.	13.	14.	15.	16.	17.	18.	19.	20.
21.	22.	23.	24.	25.	26.	27.	28.	29.	30.
31.	32.	33.	34.	35.	36.	37.	38.	39.	40.
41.	42.	43.	44.	45.	46.	47.	48.	49.	50.

1. Requires test results as soon as possible but not immediately.
   a. STAT
   b. ASAP
   c. ROUTINE
   d. TIMED

2. Requires test results (not immediately or as soon as possible).
   a. STAT
   b. ASAP
   c. ROUTINE
   d. TIMED

3. A blood draw is performed at a specific time, and test results are reported as routine.
   a. STAT
   b. ASAP
   c. ROUTINE
   d. TIMED

4. HAA stands for
   a. Hospital Acquired Anemia
   b. Hospital Associated Anemia
   c. Healthcare Acquired Anemia
   d. Healthcare Associated Anemia

5. Heel stick is performed on age
   a. 0 month to 6 months
   b. 6 months to 2 years
   c. 2 years and above
   d. None of the above

6. Venipuncture
   a. 0 month to 6 months
   b. 6 months to 2 years
   c. 2 years and above
   d. None of the above

7. Finger sticks
   a. 0 month to 6 months
   b. 6 months to 2 years
   c. 2 years and above
   d. None of the above

8. Procedure for neonatal screening using a filter paper.

a.	Fill the circle of the filter paper by touching a sufficient drop of blood to fill the circle completely. Do not touch area within the circle. Only the drop of blood should come in direct contact with the filter paper.
b.	The first drop of the blood from the heel puncture must be wiped away.
c.	Perform a heel puncture.
d.	Let it dry for recommended time frame. The filter paper must be placed horizontally when drying the filter paper.
e.	Keep the filter paper away from sunlight.

   Sequence the procedure.
   a. E, A, B, C, D
   b. C, D, A, B, E
   c. C, B, A, E, D
   d. D, C, E, B, A

9. AUTOLOGOUS is the type of blood donation; the blood may be donated by the donor for his or her use.
   a. True
   b. False

10. Donor Deferral means an individual qualified for donating blood.
    a. True
    b. False

11. BLOOD DONATION: For whole blood collection, the minimum weight of the donor should be 110 lb.
    a. True
    b. False

12. SAFETY DATA SHEET is required to be provided by the manufacturer or related entities for each hazardous chemical so that the user have information on the product they may be using.
    a. True
    b. False

13. Therapeutic drug monitoring is performed to monitor the concentrations of the drugs in the blood.
    a. True
    b. False

14. Chain of custody contains the complete paper trail of the evidence.
    a. True
    b. False

15. Blood culture is tests that are performed to detect the presence of bacteria or fungi in the blood.
    a. True
    b. False

16. NEONATAL SCREENING COLLECTION: The most basic screening includes screening for congenital hypothyroidism, galactosemia, and phenylketonuria (PKU).
    a. True
    b. False

17. Drawing an excess amount of blood from a pediatric patient can cause serious complications.
    a. True
    b. False

18. A requisition is a form a document that contains information pertaining to the patient, specimen, provider, etc. It is also known as a request form. A requisition form gives the phlebotomy technician or the professional drawing the blood the information on the type of specimen to be drawn, the type of test to be performed and other pertinent information.
    a. True
    b. False

19. Disinfecting the site of puncture is an integral step of performing the (venipuncture or dermal puncture) procedure. Post cleaning the site, allow the site to air dry.
    a. True
    b. False

20. While performing phlebotomy, if a bone is hit with either a needle or a lancet, it may cause bone infection and inflammation.
    a. True
    b. False

21. After the procedure, there may be excessive bleeding; it may be as a result of an improper technique or due to the patient having a condition that inhibits the clotting process (hemophilia).
    a. True
    b. False

22. Dermal puncture is a procedure that involves making an incision on the skin to obtain blood. The device used to create the incision onto the skin is called the "Lancet".
    a. True
    b. False

23. Anticoagulants inhibit the blood clotting (coagulation) process, thereby letting the blood collected stay in the liquid form.
    a. True
    b. False

24. Tube additive is a small proportion of an additive that is added to the tube by the manufacturer.
    a. True
    b. False

25. Butterfly needle is a specialized needle that has butterfly flaps (two) on either side with the needle placed in the center. It also has a tubing attached to the rear end of the needle.
    a. True
    b. False

26. The primary reason to identify the patient while performing venipuncture procedure:
    a. Prevent medical errors
    b. Follow standard precautions
    c. Work ethics
    d. Documentation

27. Primary reason for: Greeting the patient
    Procedure: BLEEDING TIME TEST
    a. Procedural Standard
    b. Standard Precaution
    c. Prevent Medical Error
    d. Avoid Complication
    e. Work Ethics
    f. Transportation
    g. Patients' Bill Of Rights
    h. Documentation

28. Primary reason for: Washing hands using the proper technique of hand washing.
Procedure: CAPILLARY TUBE BLOOD COLLECTION PROCEDURE
   a. Procedural Standard
   b. Standard Precaution
   c. Prevent Medical Error
   d. Avoid Complication
   e. Work Ethics
   f. Transportation
   g. Patients' Bill Of Rights
   h. Documentation

29. Primary reason for: Disposing of gloves and other supplies into their appropriate containers.
Procedure: VENIPUNCTURE USING A MULTISAMPLE NEEDLE METHOD
   a. Standard Precaution
   b. Transportation
   c. Patients' Bill Of Rights
   d. Documentation

30. Primary reason for: Applying direct pressure on incision site with a 2x2 gauze pad. Procedure: VENIPUNCTURE USING A MULTISAMPLE NEEDLE METHOD
   a. Avoid Complication
   b. Transportation
   c. Patients' Bill Of Rights
   d. Documentation

31. When performing evacuated tube collection method, the last tube must be removed before the needle is removed from the puncture site.
   a. True
   b. False

32. There are several steps involved in performing the evacuated tube collection method. Given the following steps arrange them in their proper order.

a.	With the fingers (thumb or forefinger) of the non-needle unit carrying hand, pulling the skin taut below the site of the puncture.
b.	Removing the needle and turning on (initiating) the safety device.
c.	Removing the final tube from the evacuated tube holder prior to removing the needle.
d.	Releasing the tourniquet when the blood starts to fill the initial tube.
e.	With the needle unit carrying hand, inserting the needle at an appropriate angle.

Sequence the procedure.
   a. A, E, D, C, B
   b. A, B, C, D, E
   c. E, A, D, B, C
   d. D, C, E, B, A

33. From the below-mentioned site, identify the site that is most commonly chosen to perform a bleeding time test.
   a. Antecubital crease on the palmar surface of the forearm
   b. Median cubital vein
   c. Middle finger
   d. Ring finger

34. Identify the procedure in which a reagent strip is used?
   a. Evacuated Tube Collection method
   b. Glucose testing
   c. Winged infusion set (venipuncture)
   d. None of the above

35. A vein that is not chosen to perform venipuncture are:
   a. Median Cubital Vein
   b. Cephalic Vein
   c. Basilic Vein
   d. Axillary Vein

36. Identify the procedure in which a transfer device is used?
   a. Evacuated tube collection method using needle
   b. Winged Infusion Set method using butterfly needle
   c. Syringe blood collection method using hypodermic needle
   d. Capillary tube blood collection method

37. Which of the following is not a procedural step of an evacuated tube blood collection method?
   a. Cleaning the site with isopropyl alcohol.
   b. Inspecting the needle for defects.

c. Remove a reagent strip from the reagent strip container.

d. Applying tourniquet proximal to the site of venipuncture.

38. Which of the following is not a procedural step of an evacuated tube blood collection method?
    a. Checking on the patient for hemostasis by inspecting the site of the puncture.
    b. Removing gloves using the proper technique of glove removal.
    c. Place the end (edge) of the slider slide on the drop of the blood so that the blood spreads onto the edges of the slide.
    d. Assembling equipment and supplies.

39. Which of the following is not a procedural step of a butterfly or winged infusion set blood collection method?
    a. Applying tourniquet at the appropriate location.
    b. Selecting incision site.
    c. Place the sample slide on a flat surface. Handle slides by edges only.
    d. Disposing of sharps in a sharps container.

40. Which of the following is not a procedural step of a glucose testing procedure?
    a. Disinfecting site with isopropyl alcohol.
    b. Wiping the first drop of blood and obtaining blood using a capillary tube.
    c. Uncapping the reagent strip container.
    d. Positioning the device onto the selected finger.

41. Which of the following is not a procedural step of a capillary tube blood collection procedure?
    a. Sealing of capillary tube on filling the capillary tube using a clay sealant.
    b. Applying bandage on the incision site.
    c. Placing blood onto the reagent strip.
    d. Removing gloves using the proper technique of glove removal.

42. When performing venipuncture using a butterfly needle on the dorsal of the hand, the tourniquet should be applied _____ inches above the puncture site.
    a. 2 – 3
    b. 4 – 5
    c. 3 – 5
    d. 5 – 7

43. The most common topical antiseptic used in phlebotomy procedures is the 60% isopropyl alcohol pads. The alcohol pad is mainly used to clean and disinfect the site of the puncture.
    a. True
    b. False

44. While applying the bandage on the site after the phlebotomy procedure. Ensure that the center pad is the area of the bandage that is in contact with the puncture site since the puncture site is the site that requires protection from contamination.
    a. True
    b. False

45. The syringe has two parts: The plunger and the barrel.
    a. True
    b. False

46. Coagulation is a process that causes the blood to change its form from liquid to a semisolid or gel-like substance also known as a clot. Coagulation is sometimes also known as clotting.
    a. True
    b. False

47. When performing dermal puncture for a glucose test the puncture should be made:
    a. Perpendicular to the fingerprints.
    b. Parallel to the fingerprints.

48. When performing dermal puncture on an infant heal the puncture should be made:
    a. Medial or lateral side of heel
    b. Medial side of the heel only
    c. Lateral side of the heel only
    d. Center of the heel

49. Which of the following is not the equipment or supplies that are used for performing a venipuncture using a multisample needle?

    a. Blood Collection Tube

    b. Needle Holder

    c. Reagent Strip

    d. Multisample Needle

50. Which of the following is not the equipment or supplies that are used for performing a venipuncture using a butterfly needle?

    a. Gloves

    b. Sharps Container

    c. Adhesive Bandage

    d. Capillary Tube

PRACTICE EXAM 6: ANSWER SHEET

TOTAL SCORE: <u>50</u>　　　**YOUR SCORE:** _____

1.	2.	3.	4.	5.	6.	7.	8.	9.	10.
11.	12.	13.	14.	15.	16.	17.	18.	19.	20.
21.	22.	23.	24.	25.	26.	27.	28.	29.	30.
31.	32.	33.	34.	35.	36.	37.	38.	39.	40.
41.	42.	43.	44.	45.	46.	47.	48.	49.	50.

Photo Credits

Cover angellodeco/shutterstock; 6 Apples Eyes Studio/shutterstock; 10 Centers for Disease Control and Prevention; 14 leolintang/shutterstock; 15 Luciano Cosmo/shutterstock; 22 David W. Leindecker/shutterstock; 27 Monkey Business Images/shutterstock; 34 luminast/shutterstock; 36 ducu59us/shutterstock; 37 Alila Medical Media/shutterstock; 38 TR Alila Medical Media/shutterstock; 38 MR Alila Medical Media/shutterstock; 39 Alila Medical Media/shutterstock; 40 aurielaki/shutterstock; 43 TR stihii/shutterstock; 43 LM Blamb/shutterstock; 44 TR Blamb/shutterstock; 44 B stihii/shutterstock; 45 stihii/shutterstock; 46 MR stihii/shutterstock; 47 Blamb/shutterstock; 48 Alila Medical Media/shutterstock; 49 TR Alila Medical Media/shutterstock; 49 LM Alila Medical Media/shutterstock; 49 RB snapgalleria/shutterstock; 50 stihii/shutterstock; 52 snapgalleria/shutterstock; 53 RM ducu59us/shutterstock; 53 RB Alila Medical Media/shutterstock; 54 Alila Medical Media/shutterstock; 56 stihii/shutterstock; 57 Blamb/shutterstock; 61 luminast/shutterstock; 84 angellodeco/shutterstock; 93 Thom Hanssen Images/shutterstock; 94 aurielaki/shutterstock; 101 BlueRingMedia/shutterstock; 103 TL pema/shutterstock; 103 ML Pongsak A/shutterstock; 104 IvanRiver/shutterstock; 105 Tyler Olson/shutterstock; 110 angellodeco/shutterstock; 137 angellodeco/shutterstock; 143 angellodeco/shutterstock; 155 TR Jarun Ontakrai/shutterstock; 155 MR EsHanPhot/shutterstock; 155 RB Keith A Frith/shutterstock; 161 ESB Professional/shutterstock

PRACTICE EXAM 1	PRACTICE EXAM 2	PRACTICE EXAM 3	PRACTICE EXAM 4	PRACTICE EXAM 5	PRACTICE EXAM 6
1. D	1. E	1. A	1. B	1. C	1. B
2. A	2. B	2. A	2. A	2. D	2. C
3. C	3. C	3. A	3. A	3. A	3. D
4. A	4. A	4. B	4. A	4. A	4. A
5. B	5. B	5. A	5. A	5. D	5. A
6. A	6. B	6. A	6. A	6. A	6. C
7. A	7. B	7. B	7. A	7. C	7. B
8. A	8. A	8. A	8. A	8. A	8. C
9. A	9. C	9. A	9. B	9. B	9. A
10. B	10. D	10. A	10. A	10. A	10. B
11. B	11. B	11. B	11. B	11. D	11. A
12. C	12. A	12. B	12. A	12. B	12. A
13. C	13. C	13. B	13. A	13. A	13. A
14. A	14. A	14. A	14. A	14. D	14. A
15. C	15. A	15. A	15. A	15. E	15. A
16. D	16. B	16. A	16. A	16. B	16. A
17. A	17. A	17. A	17. B	17. B	17. A
18. D	18. C	18. A	18. A	18. A	18. A
19. A	19. A	19. A	19. B	19. C	19. A
20. B	20. C	20. A	20. B	20. D	20. A
21. C	21. B	21. A	21. B	21. D	21. A
22. A	22. D	22. A	22. A	22. A	22. A
23. B	23. B	23. A	23. A	23. A	23. A
24. C	24. B	24. A	24. A	24. D	24. A
25. A	25. B	25. A	25. B	25. A	25. A
26. D	26. C	26. B	26. A	26. A	26. A
27. B	27. C	27. A	27. A	27. A	27. E
28. A	28. D	28. B	28. A	28. A	28. B
29. D	29. C	29. A	29. A	29. B	29. A
30. A	30. A	30. A	30. B	30. A	30. A
31. B	31. A	31. A	31. A	31. A	31. A
32. C	32. B	32. A	32. A	32. A	32. A
33. C	33. C	33. A	33. A	33. A	33. A
34. B	34. D	34. B	34. A	34. A	34. B
35. D	35. B	35. A	35. A	35. A	35. D
36. A	36. A	36. A	36. A	36. A	36. C
37. B	37. A	37. A	37. A	37. A	37. C
38. D	38. A	38. A	38. A	38. D	38. C
39. A	39. B	39. B	39. A	39. A	39. C
40. C	40. B	40. A	40. A	40. C	40. B
41. D	41. B	41. A	41. A	41. A	41. C
42. C	42. B	42. B	42. A	42. A	42. A
43. B	43. A	43. A	43. B	43. B	43. B
44. C	44. A	44. A	44. A	44. C	44. A
45. C	45. A	45. A	45. A	45. D	45. A
46. D	46. A	46. A	46. A	46. B	46. A
47. A	47. A	47. A	47. A	47. A	47. A
48. B	48. A	48. A	48. A	48. C	48. A
49. C	49. B	49. A	49. A	49. D	49. C
50. D	50. A	50. A	50. D	50. A	50. D

End of Chapter Review Questions Answer Key:

PHLEBOTOMY END CHAPTER REVIEW QUESTIONS (CHAPTER 1: SECTION 1)
Question Set 1: Match The Following:

D = Gloves

G = Sterilization

I = Gowns

F = OSHA

H = Contact dermatitis

C = Irritant contact Dermatitis reactions

E = Alcohol- based handrub

J = Allergic contact dermatitis reactions

A = Vehicle mode of infection transmission

B = Hypersensitivity reactions

Question Set 2: Essay Questions (Critical Thinking)

Question Set 3. Fill The Blanks:
1. Latex
2. Runny, itchy, scratchy, itchy.
3. Agent, reservoir, exit, transmission, entry, host.
4. Aerosols, sneezing, coughing, talking.
5. Infectious.

Question Set 4. Multiple Choice:
1. C
2. D
3. B
4. C
5. C
6. A

Question Set 5. True Or False:
1. True
2. False
3. False
4. False
5. True
6. True
7. False
8. True
9. True
10. True

PHLEBOTOMY END CHAPTER REVIEW QUESTIONS (CHAPTER 1: SECTION 2)
Essay Questions (Critical Thinking)

PHLEBOTOMY END CHAPTER REVIEW QUESTIONS (CHAPTER 2)
Question Set 1. Match The Following:

C = Vasodilation

E = Ventral

A = Coronal plane or frontal plane

G = Sagittal plane or median plane

J = Transverse plane or horizontal plane

B = Dorsal

H = Medial

D = Distal

F = Vasoconstriction

I = proximal

Question Set 2: Essay Questions (Critical Thinking)

Question Set 3. Fill In The Blanks
1. 55 %
2. 90 %
3. Formed elements
4. 99 %
5. White blood cells
6. Men: 4.7 to 6.1 women: 4.2 to 5.4
7. 15
8. absent, present
9. Phagocytosis
10. 30-40, 15

Question Set 4. Multiple Choice:
1. C
2. B
3. B
4. C
5. D
6. D

PHLEBOTOMY END CHAPTER REVIEW QUESTIONS (CHAPTER 3)
Question Set 1: Fill The Missing Answers
Answers can be found from page 63-73.

PHLEBOTOMY END CHAPTER REVIEW QUESTIONS (CHAPTER 4)
Question Set 1: Match The Following

F: Types of blood specimen collected

J: Gray

E: Light green or green/gray stopper

C: Light blue

G: Medial or lateral side of heel

I: Rotor

A: Types of Additives

B: Lavender tube

D: EDTA (Ethylene-Diamine-Tetra-Acetic-Acid, sodium citrate, Heparin, and sodium

H: Patients prone to develop venous Thrombosis

Question Set 2: Essay Questions (Critical Thinking)

Question Set 3: Fill The Blanks
1. **B**: Tube holder, **C**: Tube, **J**: Tourniquet
2. 2.4
3. 2.0
4. Isopropyl
5. Lab uses: chemistry, serology, immunology, and blood bank
6. Additive: SPS
7. Specimen: whole blood
8. Additive: Sodium citrate, **lab uses**: coagulation studies, PT, PTT, and fibrinogen
9. Tube: Gray
10. Tube: Gold stopper
11. Additive EDTA K2, EDTA k3, Specimen: whole blood
12. Additive: Lithium heparin and gel, lab uses: plasma determinations in chemistry studies
13. Specimen: plasma, lab uses: chemistry testing- STAT chemistry test, glucose, ammonia, and electrolytes.
14. Tube: Royal Blue
15. Specimen: serum, lab uses: STAT serum chemistries
16. Specimen: plasma, lab use: Lead.
17. K2 EDTA (potassium EDTA), Lab uses: Hematology, blood

bank, compatibility testing, and antibody screening

Question Set 4: Multiple Choice
1. F
2. G
3. C
4. D
5. G
6. D
7. D
8. B
9. D
10. D

Question Set 5: Rearrange The Information Provided In A Correct Order
1. 2, 6, 3, 5, 4, 1
2. 3, 4, 5, 6, 1, 2

Question Set 6: True Or False
1. False
2. True
3. True
4. False
5. False
6. False
7. False
8. False
9. True

PHLEBOTOMY END CHAPTER REVIEW QUESTIONS (CHAPTER 5)
Question Set 1: Match The Following
E: Inspect needle
J: Identify patient
G: Fill evacuated tubes in the correct order of draw
I: package specimen for transport
A: Verify physician's orders
C: Explain procedure to the patient
F: insert needle an appropriate angle. (15* to 30 angle)
D: Blot blood at 30 seconds interval until bleeding
B: wash hands/ don PPE

H: Remove tourniquet within 60 seconds

Question Set 2: Essay Questions (Critical Thinking)

Question Set 3: Fill The Blanks
1. Standard precautions
2. 30 seconds
3. Horizontally
4. Clay sealant
5. Downward
6. Perpendicular
7. Sharps

Question Set 4: Multiple Choice
1. D
2. B
3. B
4. D
5. C
6. C
7. B
8. D
9. A

Question Set 5: True Or False
1. False
2. True
3. False
4. False
5. True
6. False
7. True
8. True
9. True
10. True

Question Set 6: Clinical Competency Checklist (Critical Thinking)

PHLEBOTOMY END CHAPTER REVIEW QUESTIONS (CHAPTER 6)
Question Set 1: Match The Following
1. D
2. E
3. F

4. A
5. B
6. C
7. S
8. T
9. U
10. N
11. O
12. J
13. K
14. P
15. R
16. M
17. G
18. H
19. I
20. R
21. Q

Types Of Test Request (Match The Following)
1. D
2. C
3. A
4. B

Question Set 2: Essay Questions (Critical Thinking)

Question Set 3: Sequence In Order
STOOL COLLECTION IN A CONTAINER:
Write the correct number next to the step:
❖ 3,6,8,9,10,4,1,2,11,5,7
THROAT SWAB COLLECTION PROCEDURE:
Write the correct number next to the step:
❖ 7,8,6,1,2,9,5,3,4,13,14,15,10,11,12

Question Set 4: True Or False
1. False
2. False
3. True
4. False
5. False

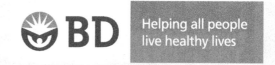

Helping all people
live healthy lives

BD Vacutainer® Order of Draw for Multiple Tube Collections

Designed for Your Safety

Reflects change in CLSI recommended
Order of Draw (H3-A5, Vol 23, No 32, 8.10.2)

Closure Color	Collection Tube	Mix by Inverting
BD Vacutainer® Blood Collection Tubes *(glass or plastic)*		
	• Blood Cultures - SPS	8 to 10 times
	• Citrate Tube*	3 to 4 times
or	• BD Vacutainer® SST™ Gel Separator Tube	5 times
	• Serum Tube *(glass or plastic)*	5 times (plastic) none (glass)
	• BD Vacutainer® Rapid Serum Tube (RST)	5 to 6 times
or	• BD Vacutainer® PST™ Gel Separator Tube With Heparin	8 to 10 times
	• Heparin Tube	8 to 10 times
or	• EDTA Tube	8 to 10 times
	• BD Vacutainer® PPT™ Separator Tube K$_2$EDTA with Gel	8 to 10 times
	• Fluoride (glucose) Tube	8 to 10 times

* When using a winged blood collection set for venipuncture and a coagulation (citrate) tube is the first specimen tube to be drawn, a discard tube should be drawn first. The discard tube must be used to fill the blood collection set tubing's "dead space" with blood but the discard tube does not need to be completely filled. This important step will ensure proper blood-to-additive ratio. The discard tube should be a nonadditive or coagulation tube.

Note: Always follow your facility's protocol for order of draw

Handle all biologic samples and blood collection "sharps" (lancets, needles, luer adapters and blood collection sets) according to the policies and procedures of your facility. Obtain appropriate medical attention in the event of any exposure to biologic samples (for example, through a puncture injury) since they may transmit viral hepatitis, HIV (AIDS), or other infectious diseases. Utilize any built-in used needle protector if the blood collection device provides one. BD does not recommend reshielding used needles, but the policies and procedures of your facility may differ and must always be followed. Discard any blood collection "sharps" in biohazard containers approved for their disposal.

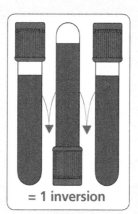

= 1 inversion

BD Technical Services
1.800.631.0174
BD Customer Service
1.888.237.2762
www.bd.com/vacutainer

BD, BD Logo and all other trademarks are property of Becton, Dickinson and Company. © 2010 BD
Franklin Lakes, NJ, 07417   1/10   VS5729-6

BD Vacutainer® Venous Blood Collection
Tube Guide

For the full array of BD Vacutainer® Blood Collection Tubes, visit www.bd.com/vacutainer.
Many are available in a variety of sizes and draw volumes (for pediatric applications). Refer to our website for full descriptions.

BD Vacutainer® Tubes with BD Hemogard™ Closure	BD Vacutainer® Tubes with Conventional Stopper	Additive	Inversions at Blood Collection*	Laboratory Use	Your Lab's Draw Volume/Remarks
Gold	Red/Gray	• Clot activator and gel for serum separation	5	For serum determinations in chemistry. May be used for routine blood donor screening and diagnostic testing of serum for infectious disease.** Tube inversions ensure mixing of clot activator with blood. Blood clotting time: 30 minutes.	
Light Green	Green/Gray	• Lithium heparin and gel for plasma separation	8	For plasma determinations in chemistry. Tube inversions ensure mixing of anticoagulant (heparin) with blood to prevent clotting.	
Red	Red	• Silicone coated (glass) • Clot activator, Silicone coated (plastic)	0 5	For serum determinations in chemistry. May be used for routine blood donor screening and diagnostic testing of serum for infectious disease.** Tube inversions ensure mixing of clot activator with blood. Blood clotting time: 60 minutes.	
Orange		• Thrombin-based clot activator with gel for serum separation	5 to 6	For stat serum determinations in chemistry. Tube inversions ensure mixing of clot activator with blood. Blood clotting time: 5 minutes.	
Orange		• Thrombin-based clot activator	8	For stat serum determinations in chemistry. Tube inversions ensure mixing of clot activator with blood. Blood clotting time: 5 minutes.	
Royal Blue		• Clot activator (plastic serum) • K₂EDTA (plastic)	8 8	For trace-element, toxicology, and nutritional-chemistry determinations. Special stopper formulation provides low levels of trace elements (see package insert). Tube inversions ensure mixing of either clot activator or anticoagulant (EDTA) with blood.	
Green	Green	• Sodium heparin • Lithium heparin	8 8	For plasma determinations in chemistry. Tube inversions ensure mixing of anticoagulant (heparin) with blood to prevent clotting.	
Gray	Gray	• Potassium oxalate/sodium fluoride • Sodium fluoride/Na₂ EDTA • Sodium fluoride (serum tube)	8 8 8	For glucose determinations. Oxalate and EDTA anticoagulants will give plasma samples. Sodium fluoride is the antiglycolytic agent. Tube inversions ensure proper mixing of additive with blood.	
Tan		• K₂EDTA (plastic)	8	For lead determinations. This tube is certified to contain less than .01 µg/mL(ppm) lead. Tube inversions prevent clotting.	
	Yellow	• Sodium polyanethol sulfonate (SPS) • Acid citrate dextrose additives (ACD): **Solution A -** 22.0 g/L trisodium citrate, 8.0 g/L citric acid, 24.5 g/L dextrose **Solution B -** 13.2 g/L trisodium citrate, 4.8 g/L citric acid, 14.7 g/L dextrose	8 8 8	SPS for blood culture specimen collections in microbiology. ACD for use in blood bank studies, HLA phenotyping, and DNA and paternity testing. Tube inversions ensure mixing of anticoagulant with blood to prevent clotting.	
Lavender	Lavender	• Liquid K₃EDTA (glass) • Spray-coated K₂EDTA (plastic)	8 8	K₂EDTA and K₃EDTA for whole blood hematology determinations. K₂EDTA may be used for routine immunohematology testing, and blood donor screening.*** Tube inversions ensure mixing of anticoagulant (EDTA) with blood to prevent clotting.	
White		• K₂EDTA and gel for plasma separation	8	For use in molecular diagnostic test methods (such as, but not limited to, polymerase chain reaction [PCR] and/or branched DNA [bDNA] amplification techniques.) Tube inversions ensure mixing of anticoagulant (EDTA) with blood to prevent clotting.	
Pink	Pink	• Spray-coated K₂EDTA (plastic)	8	For whole blood hematology determinations. May be used for routine immunohematology testing and blood donor screening.*** Designed with special cross-match label for patient information required by the AABB. Tube inversions prevent clotting.	
Light Blue / Clear	Light Blue	• Buffered sodium citrate 0.105 M (=3.2%) glass 0.109 M (3.2%) plastic • Citrate, theophylline, adenosine, dipyridamole (CTAD)	3-4 3-4	For coagulation determinations. CTAD for selected platelet function assays and routine coagulation determination. Tube inversions ensure mixing of anticoagulant (citrate) to prevent clotting.	
Clear	(New) Red/Light Gray	• None (plastic)	0	For use as a discard tube or secondary specimen tube.	

Note: BD Vacutainer® Tubes for pediatric and partial draw applications can be found on our website.

BD Diagnostics
Preanalytical Systems
1 Becton Drive
Franklin Lakes, NJ 07417 USA

BD Global Technical Services: 1.800.631.0174
BD Customer Service: 1.888.237.2762
www.bd.com/vacutainer

* Invert gently, do not shake
** The performance characteristics of these tubes have not been established for infectious disease testing in general; therefore, users must validate the use of these tubes for their specific assay-instrument/reagent system combinations and specimen storage conditions.
*** The performance characteristics of these tubes have not been established for immunohematology testing in general; therefore, users must validate the use of these tubes for their specific assay-instrument/reagent system combinations and specimen storage conditions.

Notes:

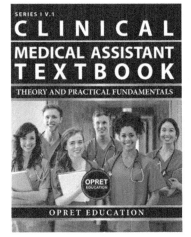
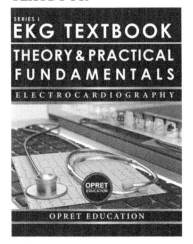
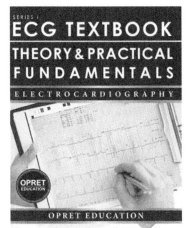
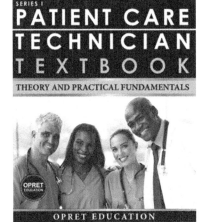
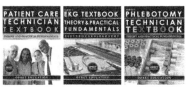
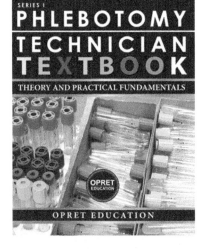
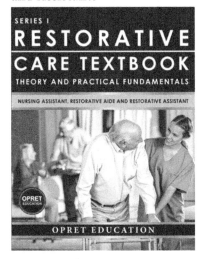